High P

THE LOST SOUL COMPANION

A Book of Comfort and Constructive Advice for Black Sheep, Square Pegs, Struggling Artists, and Other Free Spirits

"For those who feel like square pegs in a round-hole world . . . you will find ideas, wisdom, understanding and a lot of smiles in this book."

—*The Herald-Times* (Bloomington, Indiana)

"A superb little compendium of comfort and constructive advice. . . . Packed with intriguing concepts and excellent tips . . . this is a fine guide to happiness."   —*Midwest Book Review*

"Lives up to the promise of its subtitle."
—*The Dallas Morning News*

"Beautiful, whimsical, heartbreaking . . . If you are an artist or an artist-at-heart, you will love this book." —Eric Maisel, author of *The Creativity Book*

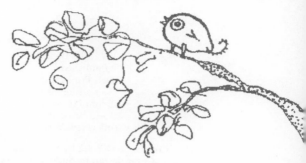

The Not-So-Lost Soul Companion

More Hope, Strength, and Strategies for Artists and Artists-at-Heart

Susan M. Brackney

Delta

A Delta Book
Published by
Dell Publishing
a division of
Random House, Inc.
1540 Broadway
New York, New York 10036

Library of Congress Cataloging-in-Publication Data

Brackney, Susan M.
The not-so-lost soul companion : more hope, strength, and
strategies for artists and artists-at-heart / Susan M. Brackney.
p.   cm.
Includes index.
ISBN 0-440-50922-X (trade paperback)
1. Conduct of life.   2. Creation (Literary, artistic, etc.)—
Miscellanea.   I. Title.
BJ1595 .B74 2002
646.7—dc21   2002019007

MANUFACTURED IN THE UNITED STATES OF AMERICA

PUBLISHED SIMULTANEOUSLY IN CANADA

October 2002
10 9 8 7 6 5 4 3 2 1
FFG

"one of the hardest things to do
is to create something from
nothing
and take it to a place where
people want
to read it or hear it
or look at it..."

– Marilyn Brackney, artist and mom

acknowledgments

Thank you Mom and Dad, Brother and
Miss Leann, and Peter for helping to
keep me strong no matter what...
Feathery pants to you, Andrew (aka Stanley P.
Mole III), for much material and editorial
support and general kindness. Thank you to
Debra Goldstein (you are actually an angel!)
and Danielle Perez, Shannon, and Shawn at
Dell...for their willingness to share their
experience and wisdom... Gustav Potthoff,
Bruce Tinsley, Tim Grimm, my mom and brother (again!),
Ben Rinehart, Lisa Gill, Rob Calder, Cathe Burris,
Steve, Paul, Michael Teague (you are going places!), Nate,
Melinda, Doug, Benjamin, the other Rob, Jeff, double J,
and the extra shy interviewees too. Also, thanks
go to Michael White, Rick Dietz, Mary Reed, Kevin
Broccoli, Bob Zaltsberg, SARK, Andrea, the reference
librarians at the Monroe County Public Library (and the
Ellettsville branch of course!) for assorted reasons...
Of course, thank you Grandma Hanna—and so many
like you—for supporting the dreamers. Finally,
Grandpa Hanna, your creative spirit surrounds us!
I am so grateful to you!

CONTENTS

THE TANGLED BLACK SCRIBBLES & OTHER PITFALLS

YAY & HOORAY!

THE APPENDIX

The Not-So-Lost Soul Companion

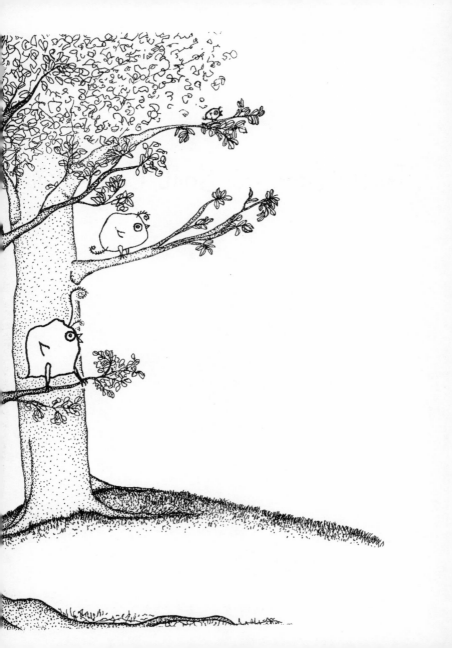

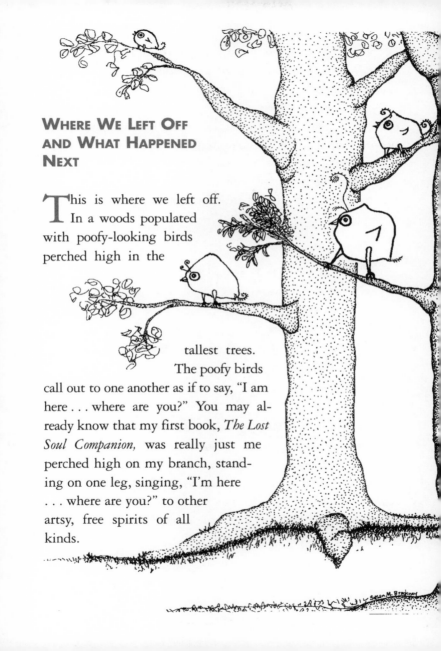

WHERE WE LEFT OFF AND WHAT HAPPENED NEXT

This is where we left off. In a woods populated with poofy-looking birds perched high in the

tallest trees. The poofy birds call out to one another as if to say, "I am here . . . where are you?" You may already know that my first book, *The Lost Soul Companion,* was really just me perched high on my branch, standing on one leg, singing, "I'm here . . . where are you?" to other artsy, free spirits of all kinds.

(Now, it's completely okay if you didn't read the first book. You can read this one and pretend there is no first book if you like and it should still make plenty of sense.)

Since then I've been able to compare notes with lots of other Lost Souls. There are many more of these intriguing people than even I had expected, and hearing from them helped me to know what to put in *this* book.

Roll out the bird translation machine and you'll hear a good deal more than just "I am here . . . where are you?"

For instance, many still struggle with depression and suicidal feelings...

"Every time I get full of really good ideas and am resolute in ambition and full of optimism, this demon keeps trying to drag me straight back into that horrible hell of inactivity, lethargy, can't-cope-ness."

"I feel like I'm fated for being a statistic of some kind or another, and it's not a good feeling. It kind of feels like I'm a ball at some carnival booth that someone is trying to win a prize with by throwing it into one of the holes. . . . Will they throw me into the hole that says suicide *or the one that says* liver disease, *or perhaps the one marked* mental breakdown*?"*

Nearly all feel like they don't quite fit...

"I feel constantly driven to think 'too deeply.' . . . I am aware to an extremely high degree that I am highly unusual. No one seems to . . . understand me. . . . I live in a very lonely world and only people like 'this' know what I am talking about."

Many Lost Souls are very ambitious...

"I want to be successful. I want to be well known. I want the whole world to know I exist. . . ."

... but no matter how hard they try it just doesn't seem like enough...

"It's like you spend all this time trying to become someone but you seem to be getting nowhere. I have dreamed of being a dancer on Broadway for as long as I can remember. Every time I feel like I might be moving up to the next level, someone is there to check my hopes and dreams at the door."

"I hold on to the frail, withering hope that I, too, am here for a worthwhile reason."

THE GROCERY-STORE EPIPHANY

Josh and I were in the snack aisle. Crinkling the bags of pretzels aside in our search for those corn chips that are shaped like small spoons. We made it all the way to the potato chips that are *baked not fried!* with no luck. Somewhere near the bright orange cheese puffs, I thought about the truck driver who had probably driven his semi filled to the top with cases and cases of this hermetically sealed goodness. I wondered what he was doing right at that moment, and I hoped he was happy.

The idealist in me likes to imagine a world full of people who are able to do what they love at least seventy-two percent of the time and still have enough to eat and a place to nap. There would be no more wage slaves, only souls who happen to get paid to do what they'd be willing to do for free.

Truck drivers like the cheese-puff guy would haul huge shipments of cola and brassieres not because they have to but because they love to—*Breaker-one-nine*. Chefs would decoratively squirt raspberry sauce on dessert plates—*Mmmm, perfect.* . . . Salesmen would sell, writers would write, doctors would doctor, painters would paint—all because they really, really want to. People would brazenly open their own flower shops—*That orchid is* Epidendrum radiatum—and because they would spend time doing what they've always wanted to do instead of what they thought they *had* to do, their endeavors succeed, they worry less, they have all that they need. It would be a world especially hospitable to artists, and that I'd love to see.

Still, that isn't exactly the epiphany I meant to tell you about. Running into Josh at the grocery store had been just what I needed that afternoon, since I'd been thinking about what to put in this book, and things hadn't seemed right. I wasn't sure why, but now I knew. This was the problem: I was about to skip right over Josh. Considering what a great guy he is, that seemed unfair.

Josh happens to be a great patron of the arts. Any extra money he has he spends on sculptures and paintings. He is himself a very creative person, and I know he could do just about anything he wanted, but I don't think he really knows what that should be.

He was a year behind me in school, and now he's twenty-seven years old. He's traveled all over and has been engaged at least twice that I know of. That day he told me he'd moved back in with his parents and was substitute-teaching high-school math. He seemed positively miserable—and Lost.

I could identify. When I began *The Lost Soul Companion* project, I had just returned from a disastrous move to California. I'd originally moved to Santa Cruz in order to pursue my art career (and to be with my boyfriend at the time . . .),

7

but it all went to hell. After that, I'd come back home and was living under a friend's loft bed. I had no job, no money, no confidence, and no peace of mind. I had been deeply depressed—at times even suicidal. I wanted to find other Lost Souls and let them know that they weren't alone.

Now that I was feeling a bit better, I was dying to leap ahead. I wanted to encourage people who already had their acts together to get on with living their dreams, but questions nagged me. First of all, do people with their acts already properly together need such help? And, secondly, how can you go from suicidal to ready-for-stardom? (And should anyone really aspire to that anyway?)

And so I decided *not* to skip all the hard parts. The truth is, I probably couldn't have written that book anyway. After all, how can someone who hasn't got her own life completely together write for the already-completely-together people? These days, I have traded in my severe depression for mild, prolonged discouragement. As for thoughts of suicide, from now on I will keep breathing—if for no other reason than to see how things turn out.

Even now, I feel about as lost as Josh was in the snack aisle. Knowing what to reach for or where to find it isn't easy.

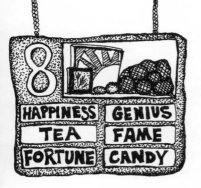

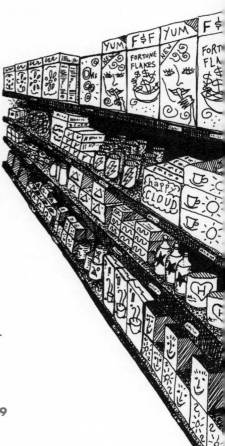

Excuse me, where can
I find Happiness?
*Do you want it in light or
heavy syrup?*
Light, I guess.
Aisle seven.
And the Fortune Flakes?
Aisle eight.

It's not, of course, like this.

9

MY HOPE FOR *THIS* BOOK

I f you're anything like me, then you live with a fairly in-
sistent urge to create and to make an indelible impression
on the whole world. There is, in my case, the small matter of
not really knowing what it is I was "meant" to do.

Truly, I never thought I would amount to anything at all.
Besides eating candy, petting animals, and taking naps, one
of my favorite things of all time is to help other creative, interesting people figure out what might make them happier.
So if I can better enable you to share your painting, music,
acting, filmmaking, or whatever it is that you live to do in
the world, then maybe I've done something worthwhile.

I've spent years trying to make a mark of my own with my
mixed-media artwork, not to mention this project too, and I
can tell you what's been working so far and what hasn't
worked at all.

I suspect you are capable of greatness. To that end, I
humbly offer some ideas to help you succeed—keep in mind,
this is my kind of success and not the kind most everyone else
thinks about. Did you make someone else happy? Did you
touch someone else with your work? *That,* to me, is success.
Are you able to spend lots of time doing what you love to do?
That is happiness. Maybe you are even able to partially—or

10

completely—support yourself with your art. *That* is true contentment.

This book is for Lost Souls looking to prepare themselves for public consumption (and, by the way, sometimes it really does feel like you've being ingested).

So I say this to you:

It's time to do Great Things...

but how?

The Dreamy Bits

TO FLOUNDER OR TO FLOURISH?

A couple of years ago I found myself sitting in a little café in Santa Cruz, California, with no job, hardly any money, and no idea what to do next. I was surrounded by successful-looking people, and I was feeling especially unsuccessful on that particular day. I drew this map of possible Future Plans:

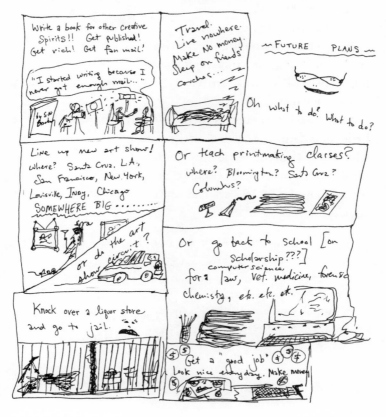

The fact that I had no idea what to do with myself was nothing new. I've always been something of a Flounder-er.

What's a Flounder-er? You know... a drifter, a rambler, a rolling stone... I wander. I float. I stray. I was undecided on a major, undecided about a career path, undecided about what to put in my grocery cart. Hesitant. Unsure. Unsettled. utterly paralyzed with possibilities and self-doubt.

Everyone flounders from time to time. Some Lost Souls are naturally flounder-y people. They may be highly creative and capable of great things, but they may also be indecisive, filled with insecurities, and very discouraged about The Future.

Here's what I wonder: Is there *really* anything wrong with a little floundering? Maybe flounder-y people are just dreamers who don't want to settle for ordinary lives. Maybe we are capable of so many great things that we can't possibly choose just one. And who said we had to make a *permanent* selection anyway?

So maybe you can choose a little something for now. Just to start with. Want to publish a book of your own poems? Direct your own short film? Have an exhibition of your paintings? Just by picking something (and it can be a really, really small thing if you like) you've already become a little Less Flounder-y!

What's the difference between floundering and flourishing? Not much, when you think about it. To flourish, you have to think carefully about what is important to you and imagine what you hope to accomplish. To flounder, you have to imagine all the ways you can fail and all the disasters you are averting by remaining completely inactive and undecided about Everything. So both require a good imagination. That means if you are good at floundering, you can be good at flourishing too! I think the first step is allowing yourself to think clearly about what you want to do and what you think you can do.

The next step is to be very, very patient, because good things take time!

A FEW FAMOUS FLOUNDER-ERS

Ralph Waldo Emerson, Agatha Christie, George Orwell, and Kevin Williamson, the guy who wrote the movie *Scream,* suggest to me that it's perfectly okay to be somewhat unstable. From others' points of view, they may have *looked* like flounder-ers, but I prefer to think that they were simply building up to their Great Flourishing.

In the case of Emerson, he spent a lot of time and energy working to become a minister, and in 1826 he began a very distinguished career in the Unitarian Church. For a few years he was very popular in the Church and he made lots of money. But after the death of his wife, Ellen, he developed serious religious doubts, and he decided to give up his min-

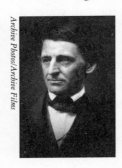

istry. Despite illness and *dispiritedness, Emerson set out for a goal he could not see,* according to biographer Robert D. Richardson in his work *Emerson: The Mind on Fire.* He left his house and sold all his furniture. For the next ten months Emerson bummed around Europe trying to collect himself. Of course, to his concerned friends and family, he looked like a Grade A Flounder-er. (Freaking out and quitting a cushy job is never easy to explain to relatives. . . .)

Richardson explained, *Emerson's new life seemed to those around him only a new failure. His family was disappointed. {His brother} Charles clucked that he had done too much "for the expression of individual opinion." Aunt Mary thought he was in dangerous waters indeed. Leaving the Second Church in Boston was a repudiation of the world of his father. Emerson was also giving up institutional affiliation and support, a guaranteed social position, and a generous and assured salary. But these same facts, from another perspective, bespeak a kind of victory, a freeing of himself from the confining forms of church and state, a chance to begin again, to live entirely—and literally—on his own terms.*

Upon his return to the United States, Emerson began lecturing and writing. In his late thirties, Emerson released his first books. It was the start of his new calling as a transcendentalist thinker. I think Emerson was just patiently evolving into what he was meant to become.

Hopefully I am too.

• • •

Agatha Christie also evolved. She had been bent on a career in music—studying singing and piano in France—

until she realized she was much too shy to perform publicly. She had never before considered becoming a writer, and even after she'd been published, she didn't see herself as a writer for a very long time. Originally, her sister had challenged her to write her first work, which was subsequently rejected by six publishers. A sev-

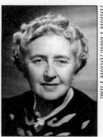

enth would accept her manuscript and, at the age of thirty, she became a published author. She wrote countless mysteries, novels, and plays, including *Murder on the Orient Express* and *The Mouse Trap,* and she has sold more books than anyone except Shakespeare.

• • •

Although George Orwell claims he always knew he wanted to be a writer, he had difficulty getting there. He hadn't had much training or experience writing, but after resigning his position as an officer with the Indian Imperial

Police, he set out to write. During the years spent refining his craft, Orwell washed dishes in Paris, taught private

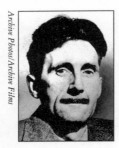

school here and there, and worked in a used-book store. When his first novels and short stories went unpublished, he destroyed them. (Imagine how this must've looked to outsiders!) Nevertheless, he pursued his creative work with a quiet intensity and independence that eventually led him to succeed with the publication of his political and literary observations and the novels *Animal Farm* and *1984*.

• • •

In the event that you think there is no hope for you at all, consider the creator of *Scream,* Kevin Williamson. His high-school English teacher told him he'd never make it as a writer, and East Carolina State University's journalism department rejected him. He studied theater instead, and, after graduating, he moved to New York City to try acting. He landed occasional bit parts, but he rarely had enough money to pay his bills. Eventually, he tried his luck on the West Coast. For a while things weren't much better there. In a 1997 *Writer's Digest* interview he recalled, *{My} phone was about to be turned off. I didn't have enough money to buy a new ink cartridge for my printer.* He now had the distinction of being a struggling actor on both coasts, but the tide was about to turn. A friend had suggested he try writing screenplays.

Williamson had always enjoyed a good slasher movie, and he got the idea for *Scream* while he was house-sitting. Alone in the house, a noise startled him. He used a cordless phone to call one of his friends, and they talked while he investigated and secured the place. But instead of offering comfort, Williamson's friend took the opportunity to terrify him just for fun. It was all the inspiration Williamson needed, and in just two weeks he wrote the screenplay for *Scream*. Ultimately he inked a twenty-million-dollar contract with Miramax, and now he continues to work on screenplays and write for television.

Sometimes appearing flounder-y to the outside world is simply part of the creative process.

A Word About Late Bloomers

It can take years and years to finally produce some of your best work. The composers Leos Janáček and César Franck achieved musical maturity in their 50s and 60s respectively. Perhaps the latest artistic bloomer of all is Anna Robertson Moses—you probably know her as Grandma Moses. She started painting in her 70s, and she painted nearly 2,000 works before her death at age 101... Do you think you're too old? There is still hope!

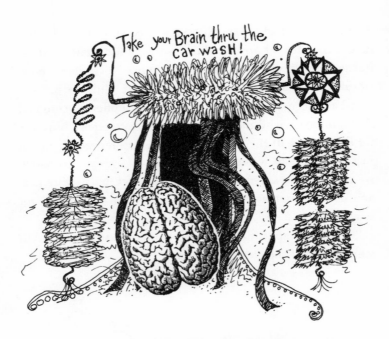

TAKE YOUR BRAIN THRU THE CAR WASH

I was terrified of the car wash when I was two. I'd try to stay calm, but anytime my parents had the misfortune of taking me through with them, I'd begin to scream hysterically, as soon as the water jets started up. My screams were so loud that they hurt my ears, but I couldn't seem to stop.

Eventually, I grew enough to be able to see over the dashboard, and then the car wash became more fascinating than frightening. Now I could silently take in the smell of surfactants creeping in along the cracks around the car doors and through the vents. Up close, the swirling reds and pinks of the mechanized scrub brushes looked like the inside of a dark, automated womb. It didn't seem so bad anymore.

These days, I don't really bother to wash my rust-bucket truck by hand, let alone go through the fancy car wash. If it were possible, though, I would pay good money to take my brain through the car wash. See, sometimes it gets so covered with gunk that I think taking it out of my skull and running it through the wash might be the easiest way to feel better.

What on Earth is Brain Gunk anyway?
    Here's my kind of gunk:
    "i'm never going to amount to anything."
    "i'm such a failure."
    "i'm a waste of perfectly good skin."

If the car-wash attendant could look away for just a minute or two, I'd let the foamy rollers cleanse away my negative thinking and the worst of my unfounded fears. Long, wiggly flaps would slap away the remains of my obsessive worrying. And then maybe a squirt of hot wax to keep my new mind-set from fading as quickly as it otherwise might.

My shiny, clean brain would be better than new. I would

be open to all kinds of wild possibilities constantly instead of just on good days. We never really know how much gunk we're carrying around in our brains until we take them—at least figuratively—through the car wash.

I've learned that Lost Souls don't need a stack of quarters to think differently about themselves and their abilities. It costs nothing to play the what-if game: *What if I played the drums? What if I swam the English Channel? What if I wrote a book?*

I never realized how many people don't let themselves dream. I think a very good job for me to have someday is that of LIFE DREAM Consultant. People would climb up some stairs to my small but cozy office full of natural light and clouds painted on the ceiling. We would talk and talk until together we figured out something that sounded like a good idea to you. Maybe you'd realize that you've always wanted to start your own marshmallow factory, and then I would help you figure out what to do next...

TOOF IS *FOOT* SPELLED BACKWARD
AND WHAT WERE *YOU* MEANT TO DO?

My Grandpa Hanna was a first-generation American and a huge dreamer. Even though he dropped out of school as a kid to help support his nine brothers and sisters, he was always talking about his ship coming in. While Grandpa was waiting for one particular ship or another, Grandma Hanna worked as an office manager at Montgomery Ward. She supported the family while Grandpa tried out all sorts of ideas.

He sang in nightclubs for a time. He sold men's clothing.

There was the grocery store that he fixed up and stocked with food. (Friends and family flocked to the store, and business would have been good—except for the fact that Grandpa didn't feel right about taking money from his friends and relatives . . . so he gave the food away.)

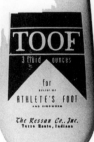

Not long after his grocery store folded, he began to design Formica tables. Formica, he said, was the material of the future. Wrought-iron bases held the bright pink Formica slabs. Grandma didn't even remember those, so I guess they must not have done very well.

Lots of people told him to go get a "real"

job. But he had already had plenty of "real" jobs. He worked construction, sold auto parts, and even worked in radio and television. I think Grandpa just preferred trying to do things his way. That and the fact that he didn't have a mentor of any sort to help guide him.

At some point he and a buddy decided to bottle and market an athlete's foot remedy called "TOOF," which, they pointed out, is *foot* spelled backward.

I hadn't actually thought of TOOF in years. One day Mom and Dad and I were in the car coming back from somewhere when Dad said, "My foot itches," and Mom replied, "Well, Larry, I think there's some TOOF in the cabinet." I love that my mom said that. She was being completely serious. Never mind that the bottle of TOOF in the cabinet was almost empty. Never mind that the concoction was very nearly thirty years old. Never mind that TOOF, a mixture of caustic acids and acetone suspended in alcohol, was a rather dangerous product even when new. Now that all the alcohol had evaporated, well, would my dad even have a foot left?

Grandpa Hanna claimed it also cured ringworm and jungle rot. Considering how the product worked, I believe him. The white plastic bottle stands about four inches tall. The directions on the back bear out TOOF's efficacy:

Cleanse and thoroughly dry feet before applying TOOF. Spray TOOF freely on affected parts night

26

and morning. After a few days, the destroyed skin will begin to peel off. Do not pick at the loose skin—allow nature to discard it. At this time, spray TOOF once daily for two or three days. Then in screaming capitals, *DO NOT APPLY ANYWHERE NEAR THE HEAD.*

A little more perseverance on Grandpa's part and maybe TOOF would be right next to the Band-Aids in medicine cabinets everywhere. But TOOF wasn't the answer.

After years and years of searching, he finally found his groove. He started his very own advertising agency and did quite well until he died of lung cancer.

Grandpa Hanna was buried on my seventh birthday. I wasn't allowed to go to the funeral because Mom and Dad thought I was too young to understand what was going on. As a result, I don't really feel like my grandpa is dead. Instead, I picture him on a tropical island, drinking fruity drinks with swords and umbrellas sticking out of them

I admire that my grandpa was a dreamer who didn't let other people discourage him. Certainly, I am grateful to Grandma Hanna for being so supportive and understanding through what must've been some very hard times. Swimming in a sea of TOOF and pink Formica tables, Grandpa might have been tempted to give it all up and settle for something more stable. Instead, he never quit trying to find out what it was that he was meant to do. And neither should we.

GUIDED BY SPIRITS: GUSTAV POTTHOFF

For all of the scads of us struggling with our creative purposes, there are still others who know exactly what it is that they are meant to do. My friend Gustav is compelled to paint feverishly colorful scenes; he cannot stop. They are payment on a promise he made to his mother a long time ago.

Gustav is one of the most resilient and amazing people I have ever known. On March 11, 1941—his eighteenth birthday—he was captured by the Japanese while serving in the Dutch army in Indonesia and forced to work on the construction of the Thailand–Burma Railway. For the next four years he worked alongside fellow Dutch, American, Australian, and English prisoners of war. In addition to deplorable working conditions and near starvation, Gustav and the others contended with scorpion bites, malaria, cholera, jungle rot, and dysentery. Thousands died—nearly one prisoner for every railroad tie, to be exact.

Gustav remembered the conditions: "We were trading always [our clothes or shoes] for sugar. Sometimes you almost naked. And the rain time, hot time! It is so humid there in the jungle, and you have to make it, [be] strong. Sometimes you wonder how many times you already dead. And still [God] says, 'It's not time for you. Wake up!' "

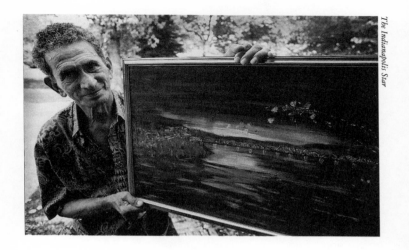

The Indianapolis Star

It was when he was stricken with cholera that Gustav made the promise he has most passionately kept. In his homeland, it is common to spiritually call out to friends or relatives for help. This is just what he did. "I called [out to] my mother and [said], 'Ma, get the Lord to help me out of this hell that I'm in . . . then I like to do something else. The story of this. Camps, prisoners, you know? This story where I been.' "

Gustav says he heard a voice that night. It told him to go to the kitchen and get hot pepper and rice. But sick men were not to be given any food. Unable to walk or stand in his condition, Gustav crawled some hundred meters to the kitchen anyway. He tells the story like this:

"I say, 'Cook, give me hot pepper and rice.'

"He say, 'No! You cannot eat hot pepper. The doctor don't like you do that.'

"I say, 'That is my last wish.'

"He say, 'Oh, that is different. I give you.'

"(If I don't say that maybe he don't give me.) He gets me a handful [of] hot pepper. It is dry pepper . . . and dry rice. I ate so much that day I think I am at a Chinese restaurant."

After his "last meal," Gustav slept and dreamed vividly. When he woke up, it seemed a miracle had happened. He could walk; he was well. Two hundred of his fellow prisoners did not survive. Ever since then he has vowed to "do something good."

But what would that be? He remembered, "I didn't know what I like to do . . . because I know no part of painting, no part of that. I never paint before. Never had the school for painting. But I promised her. . . ." As it turns out—even though he doesn't consider himself to be a painter—Gustav paints.

He paints only at nighttime when his wife is working her shift as a hospital nurse. In a small, quiet room he drips colors onto his canvases without really knowing what to expect. He explained, "I don't know how I do it. My mind [lets] me do it—my spookies."

The spookies are Gustav's spirit friends who didn't survive the prison camps. One spirit in particular—an Australian man Gustav buried along the railway—guides his hand most often. "When it's quiet, I feel something coming. I have my canvas ready a couple days before. He calls me to do it."

Details usually present themselves to Gustav the next morning. The railway, the bridge, a sunset, elephants, tools—all become very clear to him. It has been more than fifty years since his release from the prison camps, but the scenes from that time—haunting and beautiful—remain fresh.

He never sells his paintings; he only gives them away because that is what the spirits who guide his work insist upon. He said, "I paint for memory, not for the money. . . ." It is most important to him that the hardship and losses along the Thailand–Burma Railway are never forgotten. His commitment to this idea is absolutely unshakable, and I admire that. While I don't envy him his experiences, I do wish my sense of purpose were as strong as his.

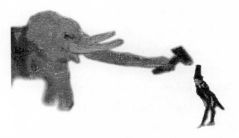

Detail from Gustav's painting Emperor, Here Is the Bill Not Paid. *An elephant punishes Japanese emperor Hirohito on behalf of POWs and comfort women alike.*

TEMPERING THE TOWERING AMBITION AND WHAT IS SUCCESS ANYWAY?

As a teenager, I actually composed a letter to *Seventeen* magazine offering my services as a glamorous fashion model in exchange for one free subscription. Not only was I not a model—had never been, in fact—but also there was the problem of my hair, my teeth, my skin. (Bad perm, crooked, and zits, respectively.) Not to mention that I had no breasts to speak of and, above all, I was much too short. Reality momentarily poked its pinky finger in my eye, and I did not mail the letter.

Nevertheless, I thought that notoriety—even fame and riches—should come to me simply because I was alive. You know, Me—the Different and Greatly Gifted One. Fortunately for everyone within three feet of me, I eventually outgrew that. It was my Towering Ambition. I had built it up so high that it nearly blotted out the sun. Its foundation was a mixture of Marshmallow Peeps and idle wishes rather than very hard work. I am lucky the whole thing didn't topple over and brain me.

I don't know exactly when or even how I dismantled the unrealistic expectations of myself, but I do know that if I hadn't I wouldn't have accomplished much of anything worthwhile yet. It's one thing to want to do great things with your life and quite another to expect the adoration of millions before you turn twenty. I admit, I used to think it would be really cool to be famous. That, I reasoned, would mean I had become a "successful" person. Now I've decided that instead of being famous it would be nice to be merely remarkable. To do that, I aim to live remarkably. For me, that means braving a nontraditional lifestyle. I've ditched the nine-to-five routine, and, mostly, I eschew material goods. And if I'm still unmarried by age eighty-five, that's okay. I'll be free to do most anything. (A nice lady I know asked me to travel with her on a medical mission to Africa to paint glass eyeballs for the villagers there. . . . Maybe I'll do that next?) I'm bound only by my physical limitations and my imagination.

My idea of success has evolved too. For me, doing creative work that is satisfying to me and also useful to others is success. Being able to at least partially support myself with my creative work is Capital S Success.

You can hope for fame and supreme wealth, but these are goals I can't encourage with an entirely clear conscience.

Let's say you do become famous. Now you are even more likely to be stalked by some whacko.

> Famous Souls who've been stalked...
> Gwyneth Paltrow, David Letterman, Steven Spielberg, Michael Landon, Clint Eastwood, Olivia Newton-John, Brad Pitt, Barbra Streisand, Kathie Lee Gifford, Jerry Lewis, Dan Rather, Madonna, Sonny Bono, Sylvester Stallone, Michael J. Fox, Michael Jackson and the list goes on...

Not to mention that you can't be too sure if your friends and acquaintances hang around because you're You or because you're Famous. You can't even go to the grocery store for tampons and milk without seeing a story in the tabloids about it the next week. (Of course, there is possibly one good thing about being famous and/or important. If there's a nuclear war, there's a small chance that some men in plastic suits will whisk you away to an underground safe haven stocked with plenty of baked beans.)

As for supreme wealth, I do think a person can have too much money. Having too much is almost as bad as not having enough, because now you have to be consumed with watching your money and keeping it safe. And what if, after you've achieved all of this, you still feel sort of empty and lost? I'd rather feel empty and lost because I wasn't famous and rich than empty and lost despite the fact that I was.

PERCEPTIONS AND MOVIE GRASS

If being merely remarkable just won't do for you, consider this: Things really aren't always what they seem to be. "Fame" and "Success" are mostly illusions mixed with lots of attitude, I think. . . .

But first, the movie grass.

My folks both worked as extras in the movie *Madison*. (In case you haven't seen it, it's about hydroplane racing in Indiana and was mostly shot on location there.) Mom and Dad were like two teenagers, getting in at all hours of the night and snickering about Crazy Bob running out of duct tape on the set.

Apparently they were to be in a funeral scene at a little country church on the outskirts of the city of Madison. It was fall and the grass around there was stiff and much too brown for the shot. A prop man came and spray-painted the grass bright green, using a long wand with a rubber hose attached to a tank full of movie-grass paint like it was just no big deal.

I think we'd find movie grass everywhere if we were willing to start looking for it. But maybe then we'd be disappointed without all of our illusions.

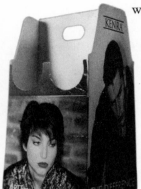

ooh-la-la!

Most of the time, things aren't really the way we perceive them to be. The glamorous girl on this Kenra mousse box looks like she lives in New York City and drinks only tall, chilled glasses of Perrier, but actually that's my friend Melinda, and she hasn't showered in two days.

"It was the middle of July, and I was moving into a new apartment and it was really, really hot," she recalled. "[The photographer] called me up and asked me if I wanted to come up and have some pictures taken, and I told him that I needed to take a shower and that I was really gross and had dandruff.

"He said, 'No, I won't be able to do it unless you come up right now.'

"I said, 'I'll come up right now, but I'm telling you I'm dirty,' and he was like, 'No, just come on up.'

"And I went up there, and I was just gross, and he said, 'Man, you *do* have dandruff!'

"So he just put lipstick on me. He didn't put anything in my hair. He just took a picture of me exactly the way I came in there—that was the cover of the mousse box."

Melinda is not even a professional model. Her hairstylist happened to ask her once if she'd like to do some modeling, and that's how she originally met the photographer who shot the dirty Melinda pictures. Some of her pictures have even ended up in national hairstyle books!

While she enjoyed the opportunity, modeling just isn't what Melinda lives to do. She admitted, "I had one of my friends get really angry with me for not deciding to go to New York or to LA and try my way with things. . . . I'm not going to put time into putting shit together and trying to sell my face. That just doesn't sound cool to me." Since she is a greasy-haired model who isn't really a model, I consider Melinda to be accidental movie grass.

Some people try to turn themselves into movie grass on purpose. They want to be perceived as famous or successful and so they act that way long before they have fully become either one. I heard that David Bowie stopped opening doors for himself fairly early in his career. He wanted to be treated like a rock star, so he began acting like a rock star—and this meant making sure someone else was always around to get the door for him. It must've worked.

Just starting out, the actor George Hamilton rented a Rolls-Royce to drive around in to help his image. Upon seeing the lifestyle to which he was supposedly accustomed, one movie's producers decided they certainly couldn't pay him scale, so they gave him a raise.

Do I condone the fake-out? Nope. I'm not telling you about the on-purpose movie grass so that you, too, can milk other people's faulty perceptions of you for all they're worth.

No. I just want to point out that our collective sense of reality is often being manipulated—and sometimes we are unwitting accomplices to our own deception!

DUELING BANJOS AND THE WHEEL OF CREATIVE WILL

I almost gave up writing this book completely. It was right after I finished reading Dave Eggers's book *A Heartbreaking Work of Staggering Genius,* which, by the way, it was. When I compared my abilities to Dave Eggers's, I decided that I'd only been *playing* at writing and that I didn't have anything really important to say.

Just so you know, I keep a flashlight, a pen, and the crossword puzzle under the covers with me at night. Usually I don't manage to fill in even one six-letter word before my eyes get droopy and I click the flashlight off. Okay. So, I didn't realize it, but Dave Eggers had really gotten to me. I even had a dream about him, and it happens that my empty crossword puzzle came in handy. I scrawled the whole dream on the folded-up newspaper. This is exactly what I wrote:

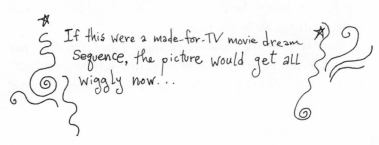

If this were a made-for-TV movie dream sequence, the picture would get all wiggly now...

Dave Eggers was lying on the floor
of his home. Naked. Dripping candle wax on
himself—his nipples mostly. It hurt me just watching
him. And I couldn't see him very well. It was
as if I were looking through the pinhole part
of one of those pinhole cameras which is really
just a box with a tiny hole poked in it. Inside
the box would be my eyeball—the optic nerve
all coiled up inside but still offering me some
visual information nonetheless. I am telling my
boyfriend that I have heard that Mr. Eggers is
a very remote person. _Ain't no one gettin' in
there._

   Mr. Eggers has also drawn little dashes and
numbers all over his waistline with a black
marker—kind of like Buffalo Bill from _Silence of the
Lambs._ Like he's going to make pants out of himself
while he's still in his own skin.

   Anyway, my boyfriend says, are you interested
in him? And I say to him, well, that would certainly
be inappropriate. I'm with you! And he says,
so you are interested! And I say, yeah, maybe
a little—even though in real life I don't
think of Mr. Eggers in this way, have never
even met the guy.

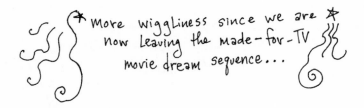

More wiggliness since we are now leaving the made-for-TV movie dream sequence...

I had no idea he was hanging around in my subconscious. How did he get in there? When had I let him in? Maybe it was all those jelly beans I'd had before bed. I had, after all, gone to sleep thinking only of quilts.

I realized then that sometimes it's hard to really understand the negative influence other artists' works can have on us. While some creative people feel very hopeful and inspired when they read a great book or hear a new band, others are devastated that they didn't write that novel first or that their band doesn't have as incredible a sound. Not many people will admit to that, of course. After all, who wants to seem jealous and pathetic? Inconsequential or inept? (I certainly don't, but sometimes I can't help but feel like a glorious loser!)

I started to feel better about all this after I learned about Brian Wilson of the Beach Boys. Much better, in fact. It seems that the Beach Boys and the Beatles were sort of like dueling banjos in the sixties. Author Timothy White explains in *The Nearest Faraway Place: Brian Wilson was taking cues from the Beatles. The Beatles were taking cues from the Byrds, who were taking cues from the Beach Boys, the Beatles, and Bob Dylan.*

Both the Beatles and the Beach Boys were on Capitol Records, and the company's attention was divided not altogether equally between them. *To Brian's ego, the Beatles' challenge represented a fight to the death,* according to author Steven Gaines in *Heroes and Villains: The True Story of the Beach Boys.*

Gaines added that Brian Wilson told a journalist at the time, *"When I hear really fabulous material by other groups, I feel as small as the dot over the* i *in 'nit.' Then I just have to create a new song to bring me up on top. . . . That's probably my most compelling motive for writing new songs—the urge to overcome an inferiority feeling. . . . I've never written one note or word of music simply because it will make money . . . and I do my best work when I am trying to top other songwriters and music makers."*

This seems like a pretty good attitude and, for a while, it seemed to be working for him.

When the Beatles released *Rubber Soul* in December of 1965, they broke all the existing sales records for an album by selling 1.2 million copies in just nine days. They were more widely received than the Beach Boys had ever been, and Brian Wilson was determined to make a *complete statement* with his next album. He set out to *make the greatest rock-and-roll album ever made.*

He slaved over *Pet Sounds,* which was released in 1966. Indeed, it is an excellent album—especially when you consider the limitations of the recording technology of the time. Maybe it was ahead of its time. Or maybe it was the fact that Capitol was a bit timid with its promotion of *Pet Sounds*. For whatever reason, the album fizzled commercially. Afterward, White writes, *Brian Wilson settled back into his Laurel Way lair, crushed by the commercial anticlimax of* Pet Sounds *but determined to distract himself with the insular creative realm he had conjured.* Wilson conceptualized a new album to be called *Smile,* but Capitol Records eventually abandoned the project because he just couldn't seem to finish what he'd started. Wilson's use of drugs and his inability to get along with friends and family didn't help matters. I doubt they meant to, but the Beatles finally pushed him over the edge.

Gaines explained, *Two new Beatles singles, "Penny Lane" and "Strawberry Fields," {were} so wondrous and different-sounding that Brian was crushed.* He continued, *When Brian finally heard* [Sergeant Pepper's Lonely Hearts Club Band], *he was shattered. The greatest album in the history of rock-and-roll had already been recorded.*

In place of *Smile,* Capitol Records hastily slapped together *Smiley Smile,* which ultimately amounted to a slap in the face to die-hard Beach Boys fans. (Sometimes I worry that *The Not-So-Lost Soul Companion* will be just another *Smiley Smile,* even though I am trying to make *Smile.*)

Brian Wilson still makes music, but not quite like he used

to. I think something sort of broke in him, and I can understand that. At least I'm not the only one to feel discouraged—even paralyzed—by others' great works. Some people do choose to give up completely, but others are only out of commission for a short while. That's the case with Mike Bloomfield, a blues guitarist who performed with the Paul Butterfield Blues Band. He told *Guitar Player* magazine about seeing Jimi Hendrix play for the first time: *"Hendrix burned me to death. I didn't even get my guitar out. H-bombs were going off, guided missiles were flying. . . . He just got right up in my face with that axe and I didn't even want to pick up a guitar for the next year."*

This phenomenon is not limited to musicians either. My painter friend Michael Teague told me that Picasso's father, don Jose, quit painting completely after he saw his son's first painting. The story is substantiated in *The Success and Failure of Picasso* by author John Berger, who writes: *Picasso's father was a provincial art teacher, and, before his son was fourteen, he gave him his own palette and brushes and swore that he would never paint again because his son had out-mastered him.* It makes for a good story, but, happily, it's not entirely true. According to biographer John Richardson, Picasso exaggerated about all sorts of things—this story included.

In his book *A Life of Picasso,* he explained, *Some small incident seems to have been magnified by Picasso . . . and taken much too seriously by one credulous biographer after another—ultimately by the artist himself.* We do know that Picasso's father wasn't a great painter, that his eyesight was failing, his hands were shaky, and his work wasn't particularly well received. He had been devastated by the loss of his daughter to diphtheria, and I'm sure watching Picasso excel at such an early age didn't help either, but in the face of all that, I think it is very compelling that, as Richardson puts it, *{don Jose} went on wielding his feeble brush until well into the twentieth century.*

Maybe painting was like breathing for don Jose. Maybe it was such a habit that he couldn't bear to stop. Perhaps he fell in love with the creative process and that is why he was able to continue despite living under the same roof with a genius. If he could keep painting, I guess I can keep writing.

And if there is such a thing as a Wheel of Creative Will—and there is, since I just made it up—then a guy like Picasso's dad isn't anywhere on it. Neither is my friend Kita, a tattooist who feels "totally inadequate looking at a Jack Rudy tattoo." She says, "When you have to feed and house six kids, you tend to just keep on working despite the fact you don't feel as good about your work as you should. So I just [keep] at it. Now I just don't look at anyone else's work. . . . I judge myself against myself and appreciate any improvements I can see."

For all the people left who might get really discouraged by others' works, here is the Wheel of Creative Will:

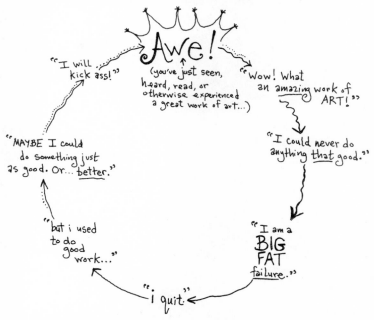

Some people get stuck at "I quit" for all time. Some people get stuck there for just a while. Me, I think I am permanently at "Maybe I could do something just as good . . ." even though it might be healthiest not to be stuck on the silly wheel at all.

Instead of comparing myself to the estimable Dave Eggers—or anyone else, while I'm at it—I'm going to try to compare my creative work to my own past efforts. Maybe then the bad dreams will stop.

Hard Work

&

Many Twisty Roads

THE RIGHT REASONS AND THE "MAN WAY" VS. THE "WOMAN WAY"

Before you ever roll up your sleeves, I hope you will make sure you're doing things for the right reasons. I say that doing something solely for money is not a good reason. The need for overwhelming public recognition is no good either.

There are filmmakers who care more about grossing millions of dollars than producing heartfelt films. There are musicians who would stop at nothing to make it to Number One on *American Top 40*. Many of them have become so product-oriented that they seem to have little regard left for the creative process itself. The filmmakers in question may have no emotional attachment to their projects. The same goes for the musicians. It's the same with everyone creating for the wrong reasons.

My friend Paul and I have gone around and around about this. He says there's nothing wrong with being very product-oriented. The real problem, he says, is being too *process*-oriented. Whether it's a problem or not, most of us *are* much more process-oriented. We paint, write, sculpt, etc., because we live to create; we enjoy the process. If we're able to sell the works we so lovingly produced, that's all the better.

Paul, on the other hand, is all product. He's a novelist who finds his market long before he bothers to begin a new manuscript. He doesn't write because he loves to write. He writes because he wants to make Stephen King kind of money. To that end, he'll study his intended audience carefully—examining its likes and dislikes, wants and needs, hopes and dreams, and then and only then will he put pen to paper. He says he has completely taken his own ego out of the writing process.

His way of doing things used to horrify me, but I understand it a little better now. (Now, don't get mad about this part; I think it's sort of interesting. . . .) Paul says there's a "man way" to do things and a "woman way." "Women form relationships with things. Men conquer things," he says. The man way is calculating, goal-oriented, and logical. Paul's novels are deliberately crafted for a specific demographic, but, he notes, that shouldn't be detectable in the finished product. The woman way is less structured and more emotionally significant to the creator.

This is all a little too black and white for me, but if I had to pick, I'd say I'm in the woman category for sure. Still, I wonder if a person couldn't have "man" qualities *and* "woman" qualities working together instead of all of one and none of the other. I do see value in mixing some man parts in with the woman way. My friend Mike pointed out that Paul's way of doing things can be useful during certain parts of a project. He said that everyone needs a coherent plan and a good sense of their respective audience. Nevertheless, I must add that if you buy into that "man way" one hundred percent of the time, then you're reading the wrong book.

Here's why: I think it's important to ask ourselves a slew of questions about what we're doing to make sure our hearts are in the right place. For instance, will your project benefit other people besides just you? Does it make a positive impact in the lives of others? Do you feel strongly about your creative work? Do you live to do it? Do you think about it even when you're not working on it? Do you get excited about it? Does it make you happy?

Also, would you do your project if there were no possibility that you'd make lots of money from it? Would you do it if there were no chance that you'd become famous? Would you do it if there were no chance that you'd win any kind of awards or public recognition?

If the answers are yes, yes, a thousand times yes, good! These are fine indicators that one's heart *is* thumping away in the right place. Now, how strong is your resolve? Can other people easily talk you out of doing your creative work? If they can, maybe your project really isn't that important to you after all. On the other hand, if you're unwavering in your devotion, wonderful. Because you're going to need all of your good reasons and your resolve—especially when things go wrong. And if other people tell you, "It won't work" or "It's not a good idea," you'll be able to persevere because you'll have the strength of your own convictions rather than idle hopes for money, public recognition, fame, and who knows what else.

I think if you have genuine feeling for your work, it shows, and many good things will come to you naturally. I also happen to think that if you're faking it, people will know.

FALL DOWN SEVEN TIMES, STAND UP EIGHT

Fall down seven times, stand up eight" is a Japanese proverb I first came across at my "real" job. Someone in middle management was handing out these little cards with various uplifting sayings printed on them. I still have mine. Even though I thought the idea of some corporation printing up slick inspiration cards to keep the plebes motivated was kind of gross, I decided to overlook the messenger and focus on the message instead: Fall down seven times, stand up eight.

If you look into the past of any accomplished soul, you will find failures. William Faulkner was a disappointing poet long before he turned to prose. Actor and screenwriter Billy Bob Thornton was a frustrated rock musician. Steven Spielberg was a high-school dropout.

Our failures aren't always the result of simple ineptitude. Sometimes the shortsightedness of others is at least partly to blame for our setbacks. An official from Decca Records told manager Brian Epstein that the company didn't want to record his band, the Beatles. Epstein said, "He told me they didn't like the sound. Groups of guitars were on the way out." The *San Francisco Examiner* once sent a rejection letter to Rudyard Kipling, telling him that he didn't know how to use the English language.

Other times our *own* shortsightedness is to blame. For instance, Gary Cooper rejected the leading role in *Gone With the Wind,* saying, "I'm just glad it'll be Clark Gable who's falling on his face and not Gary Cooper."

I doubt he had access to those uplifting cards, but Samuel Beckett wrote, *Try Again. Fail Again. Fail Better.* The poor man should know. His existence was peppered with mental breakdowns, uncertainty, rejection, and, yes, failure. And yet he persevered. I suspect that many former "failures" were able to persevere in the face of adversity because they were very committed to their work and they had faith in their own abilities—even when others didn't.

Can you imagine organizing your own tours and playing out night after night steadily for six years without having landed a decent record deal? That's just what the Beatles had to do. And Cyndi Lauper would struggle as a vocalist for ten years before her hard work would pay off.

Sometimes, no matter how hard you work, or for how long, the opportunities still don't come. George Bernard Shaw said, "The people who get on in this world are the people who get up and look for the circumstances they want and, if they can't find them, make them." Sometimes it is necessary to make opportunities for yourself—or at least start looking for them in unusual places.

I once saw an artist sitting on his porch with a row of bright acrylic paintings propped against his house. A sign read: ORIGINAL ARTWORK FOR SALE. You've got to start somewhere!

Aspiring authors can self-publish or even look into print-on-demand if they don't want to risk too much.

Untested playwrights can organize free, public performances in local parks to get exposure and feedback.

When Sting couldn't get his song "Desert Rose" on radio stations or MTV, he licensed the rights to Jaguar, which used his video in a television commercial. The deal made him big bucks, and the exposure helped get Sting's song—and subsequently his latest album—the attention music-industry giants previously denied it. *New York Times* reporter John Leland explained: *In theory, commercial licensing gives musicians a way around the gatekeepers of the music business. Musicians traditionally need record companies to manufacture, distribute and promote their work. . . . Licensing, in turn, can provide operating money and blanket exposure—through commercials, film and television soundtracks, even toys and video games. This means freedom not just from record companies but also from the boundaries of radio and MTV.* A musician named Richard Hall (you know him as Moby) got his start this way. Maybe you could too.

With the availability of CD burners and MP3s, it's a pretty good time to be an independent musician. While I haven't dabbled with those things just yet, many of my more technologically advanced friends have. My own brother told me this about a distant acquaintance in Chicago: "She's sort of a one-woman band. It's kind of a Goth, Dead-Can-Dance kind of thing. We went and downloaded some songs of hers off MP3.com, and they were really great and we bought her CD. We've actually bought several CDs from her, and she was really delighted. She's just one person plus some mixing engineers she happens to know. Now, a couple of years ago, how would anyone ever have heard her music? No one would've, and it just would've been a dream. The ability to realize that dream is much more real now."

In general, the Internet is a great equalizer. Anyone with access to a good public library can share his original artwork, writing, music—whatever—via the Internet with the whole world!

But what if you try to go through the back door and you *still* fail? Consider what authors Carole Hyatt and Linda Gottlieb have to say in their book *When Smart People Fail: It is important to understand what failure is . . . and what it isn't. Success and failure are not polar opposites; they are parts of a con-*

tinuum. One can lead to the other with great ease. Neither is likely to be permanent; the irony is we believe both will last forever. They continue, *If you are fully involved with what you do and feel that you have done it as well as you can, there can be no lasting feeling of failure.*

LANA THE LUCKY

There are some people who believe that success is just a matter of being in the right place at the right time. (Once in a great while, that's true.) These are the same people who love the story of Lana Turner's discovery. She and her mother had moved to Hollywood from Idaho, hoping to find better job prospects. Not long after, the publisher of the *Hollywood Reporter* plucked Lana from obscurity as she sipped a Coke at the Top Hat Café. She was only fifteen. Of her discovery and long career she once said, "If I could have foreseen everything that was going to happen to me, all the headlines my life would make, all the people who would pass through my days, I wouldn't have believed a syllable of it!" Turner made over fifty films and did live theater and television too. And, sure, this is a great story, but most opportunities don't present themselves quite so easily these days. Try to find a soda fountain, for starters, then sit there for hours sucking down Cokes if you don't believe me.

→ Did you know that Lana Turner shaved her eyebrows off for the movie "The Adventures of Marco Polo"? The movie makers wanted her to have straight black ones instead of her real eyebrows, and, after the movie was done, they never grew back. (Is that the price of fame?...)

Maybe you look great in tight blue sweaters, but that doesn't mean you'll be the next Lana Turner. (And is losing your eyebrows really worth it?)

It's perfectly natural to want to be noticed or recognized for something on a reasonable scale, but without a solid plan—and the right frame of mind—you probably won't be.

EXCUSES, EXCUSES

My mom used to say something to me that made me crazy. Whenever I'd tell her I didn't think I could accomplish something or other, she'd yell, "Don't tell me why it won't work! Tell me how to *make* it work!" At the time I didn't know why it infuriated me so much, but now I do.

Her tiresome statement put all of the responsibility back on me. It meant I had to go back to the drawing board and that I would actually have to do work. Now I find myself saying it all the time.

When faced with difficulty or what seems like an insurmountable obstacle, so many people just seem to want to give up. They so quickly say, "Oh, I could never do that." Or, "That'll never work." I still say those things sometimes, but I try not to since there are plenty of negative people in the world already.

I do my best to start every project like I'm going to finish it no matter what happens. (That's not to say I don't have stacks and stacks of unfinished projects lying around—but I fully intend to get to them one of these days.)

Before I even bother to plan a project—such as this book that you are holding right now—I make sure I believe the project is worth doing and then I commit to finding a way to make it work. Of course, sometimes I've been known to work against myself. . . .

WHY SHANNON ESTES KICKED MY ASS

It was the third-grade creative-writing contest. My entry was a fine selection of short stories—some of my best work at the time—including "The Duck That Could Not Swim," "The Cat Who Would Not Talk," "The Skunk That Had No

Scent," "The Wind That Could Not Whistle," and, of course, "The Frog That Had No Skin."

5.
ONCE THERE WAS A HAPPY FROG WHO HAD NO SKIN. HE HAD NO SKIN BECAUSE HE ESCAPED FROM BIOLAGY CLASS. HE TIED RUBBER BANDS AROUND HIS BODY TO KEEP HIS PARTS FROM FALLING OUT ON THE GROUND. THAT DAY HE WAS JUST HOPPING AROUND, WHEN A BOY WHO WAS PICKING HIS NOSE AT THIS TIME PICKED UP THE FROG NAMED FREDDY, UP. FREDDY WAS TERRIFIED! SUDDENLY HE WAS TAKEN TO A BUILDING, THEN HE REMEMBERED WHY THAT'S THE SAME PLACE I ESCAPED FROM. THEN HE WAS TAKEN TO THE SAME ROOM IT SAID BIOLAGY ON THE DOOR. HE WAS TAKEN TO A ROOM AND KILLED. THE BOY GOT AN A ON HIS TEST ANYWAY BECAUSE ALL HIS PARTS WHERE STILL IN HIS BODY. THE MORAL OF THIS STORY IS: IF YOU DON'T HAVE ANY SKIN BE SURE TO TIE RUBBER- BANDS AROUND YOUR SELF SO YOUR PARTS WON'T FALL OUT ON THE GROUND.

I could tell you that they were carefully crafted tales of loss and self-discovery, but I'd be lying if I did. Really, they were just morbid little vignettes designed to shock and delight my classmates.

The whole class got to vote for their favorite entry, and I would've been a shoo-in for first place were it not for Shannon Estes—the most popular girl in my class and my on-again, off-again nemesis. I don't even remember what her story was about, but I do remember that I voted for her work because I thought it *had* to be better than mine simply because it had been written by *the* Shannon Estes. And, besides, it wouldn't have been right to vote for my own story, would it?

I lost by one vote.

If I had just voted for myself I would've won, but my own lack of confidence held me back. It's funny what we remember from the past. (Shannon, are you out there? What was your story about again? And, I must know, you didn't vote for me, did you?)

She was a shrewd competitor, and I could've learned a thing or two from her if I'd thought about it. Early on, she won the affections of Steve Gillespie—a real dreamboat I'd always had my eye on. She even called me at home one night to tell me that she was "going to beat the pants off me in the spelling bee tomorrow." She had rattled me (I was even more easily rattled back then), and I fouled up on the word *least.* I spelled it *L-E-A-S-E-D* because I forgot that the other word even existed. Do you ever do that?

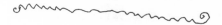

Sadly, my lack of self-confidence endures (but it's not quite as bad as it once was). You'd think getting a book deal with a division of Random House would help, wouldn't you? It didn't. In the process of trying to help other Lost Souls succeed, I *did* have some success of my own, but the truth is, when I got my book deal I felt like a big faker. Like I had fooled my agent and all the editors into publishing my talentless dreck. Worse yet, they were willing to publish this sequel! Ever the optimist, I figure now I can potentially fail on a global level. If my experience is any indication, it looks like even when you do succeed at something, the niggling doubts and fears never really go away. Negativity may be around every corner, but we just have to keep moving on anyway.

YOU MIGHT BE WHAT YOU THINK YOU ARE

Accrording to Carole Hyatt and Linda Gottlieb in *When Smart People Fail*, *To be committed—indeed, to be successful at anything—you have to believe you can do it. You must be able to picture yourself as successful. It is that picture, an internal model of success, that allows you to "disturb the universe" to accomplish your goal.*

This is not a new idea—even the Greek Stoic philosopher Epictetus believed it: *First, say to yourself what you would be; then do what you have to do.*

Hyatt and Gottlieb tell of meeting two creative souls with very different attitudes: *Recently we talked with two young men, both a few years out of college, both talented writers, and both waiting on tables to pay their bills. John, the first young man, described himself by saying, "I'm a waiter." Barney, the second fellow, said, "I'm a writer, working as a waiter." Both were writing, but John labeled himself a waiter; Barney labeled himself a writer. When we asked in some detail what each of them was actually doing, it came as no surprise that John, the "waiter," was writing only a few pages a week, while Barney, the "writer," was working systematically every day. In other words, the self-labeled "writer" was behaving like a writer, and the self-labeled "waiter-who-hoped-to-be-a-writer" was acting exactly like the unclear label he had given himself. "A rose is a rose is a rose," and, like the rose, all of us behave according to what we say we are.*

That sounds pretty good, but it's not always true. I told my writer-friend Paul the waiter/writer story, and he said the only thing that he can be sure of is that one guy is boastful and the other guy is modest. He said only a comparison of their writings can be useful and that maybe the "waiter" struggles with every word—crafting "tiny diamonds" in private—whereas the "writer" is a hack. Maybe. Of course, maybe Paul was being a little defensive since he is a writer of the tiny-diamond variety.

It is one thing to *say* you are a This or a That. And quite another to truly *be* a This or a That. Paul knows one "writer" who never writes anything. Instead, he smokes a lot, drinks a lot, and criticizes television and society a lot. Although he may have a good start on the stereotypical writer's lifestyle, he is no writer.

Similarly, you'll have to do more than carry around a pair of drumsticks to be a drummer. (Of course, if all you really want is to *look* like a drummer, then that's not a bad start.) It seems to me that you won't get anywhere just hoping for success, but combining a hopeful attitude with hard work will take you at least part of the way there.

Cathe Burris and Dispensing with Fear

I have known Cathe Burris nearly my whole life. When I was five or six, Cathe and my mother would run into each other at an art show or the local art-supply store and then would talk for an eternity while I examined their knees and shoes and wanted very badly to go home and play with my pet feather. Now that I'm much

Heather the Feather was beautiful, Barbie pink. She lived in a pickle jar. I even made her her very own toothbrush.

older and somewhat taller, I can really appreciate all of Cathe. We have conversations of our own, and she has taught me a lot about being Uncontainable—a very important quality for everyone hoping to support themselves primarily with their creative work—and dispensing with big, bad fear.

What's UNCONTAINABLE?

Being uncontainable means you don't have to allow yourself to be pigeonholed. You don't have to be only a "serious" painter or only a "dedicated" actor or only a "groundbreaking" playwright . . . and there is really no shame in being open to any opportunity which presents itself.

I freely admit that a woman once came to me with a pillow from her sofa. She commissioned a painting from me which would accent her "colors" perfectly, and I rose (or sank depending on your point of view) to the occasion because I really needed the money.

Partly because she needed the money and partly because she just happens to enjoy learning new things, Cathe has been very open to all sorts of opportunities for the past twenty-three years. Besides being a fine painter, Cathe has a very technical graphic-arts career too. She has created her fair share of logos and has painted lots of signs. She's even done race-car lettering! She explained, "I didn't want to say, 'Oh,

I'm just a painter. I only want to paint.' I was open to learning new skills, which always opens doors. I wasn't a prima donna."

Maybe she would rather have earned all of her income by selling her original artwork, but Cathe knows that isn't the easiest thing to do. "We all know that only a small percentage of the population is even going to *buy* original art. There are all these things that are chipping away at your so-called success," she said. Nevertheless, Cathe sold many of her original works. So many, in fact, that she had become a little afraid to change her painting style. Somehow, she'd managed to pigeonhole herself as a painter of "pretty dreamism"—lots of muted landscapes done in fanciful pastel tones.

Something terrible would happen before she would be able to take herself out of that particular pigeonhole: Cathe was diagnosed with breast cancer. "There was a lot of fear going on. There was a lot of sadness . . . and so that's what came out of my work," she recalled.

Cathe replaced the pastel pinks and purples of her past with dark colors and sometimes disturbing imagery.

"I felt like a truer me was coming out. That I was finally—maybe for the first time—allowing myself to be truly honest with my art."

But sometimes change has its price. Cathe said, "I would have clients that I had sold work to before say, 'Oh, can I come out to your studio and see your new work?' and I'd say, well, sure, and it was very uncomfortable for them and for me. [These new paintings] were my emotions, and I understood from a business standpoint that people would not want to hang my emotions over their couches. They would want pretty paintings. Comfortable paintings. Paintings that they could relate to."

Sadly, her art sales were no longer brisk. And then came the negative comments. Cathe's patrons told her that the new work frightened them. "I had people say, 'You must be terribly sad.' And I wasn't. I had somebody say, 'When are you going to go back to your pretty things?' I said probably never. It's a permanent change.

"That time made me question even myself about what I was doing. When I saw that I wasn't going to go back to [the old style], then I really questioned why I [had been doing that work] to begin with. Was I doing it for money? Was it the pats on the back after you sell something? . . . It made me question a lot of things." I am grateful that Cathe was able to beat her cancer—and that she's so Uncontainable.

Her painting style has continued to evolve, and I continue to learn a lot from Cathe. She says Lost Souls should never limit their career choices or be afraid to experiment with their creative work. "Something happened to me that made me say, 'Hey! I want to experience things!' I was afraid to fly. Now I fly. I was afraid to change my art. My art changed. Nothing happened. Many more things have come to me by a willingness to say, I don't have to be who I thought I was or who people thought I was." Amen.

MOANY, MOANY . . . STEADY JOBS, SHIT JOBS

My friend Limbozo says he sometimes thinks he's not really being who he was meant to be. He explained, "I work hard every day at a decent job. It's not what I want to be doing, but it's really not so bad either." In his spare time he's a musician and a songwriter, but keeping things in balance isn't easy. "[There] are . . . times that I imagine myself cutting everything loose. Where I think about dropping everything and running off to Paris or riding across the country on a motorcycle. I . . . long for chaos. I have dangerous notions at times. But I know that I need this life as it is in order to fulfill my creative needs. I have starved before. I don't think I was any more creative at the time than I am now."

I can relate. Working a steady day job for more than six months makes me feel like a pent-up cockroach. (I realize putting this in print won't help my future employment prospects, but will any perky human-resources types really read this book anyway?)

Here's something nuts: To get out of going to work at a waitressing job, I once seriously considered breaking my own arm—the left one since I am right-handed. I didn't want to wait tables even one more subservient day, and I figured they wouldn't make me if my whole left arm were stuck in a cast.

Partly, I was sick of Chili Man. He was a small man with

shiny, dyed black hair who came in at seven P.M. every day to order a bowl of chili with extra crackers and a glass of water, no ice. He always sat at the same booth in my section and left cracker crumbs everywhere. It wasn't that I had anything in particular against him, but the predictability of it all—not to mention the smell of bleach water—was wearing on me.

Evading my desk job would require more serious injuries. While I was a library circulation clerk, I considered running my car off the road or, worse, swerving into oncoming traffic just to have some extra free time. I realize other people just feign illness for a day or two, but I am much too honest for that. I could've just made myself throw up so I could call my boss and say, "I just threw up," but that never occurred to me until just now.

The job itself wasn't bad. The people were really nice and the work was pretty easy,

I even got to be a fairy once!

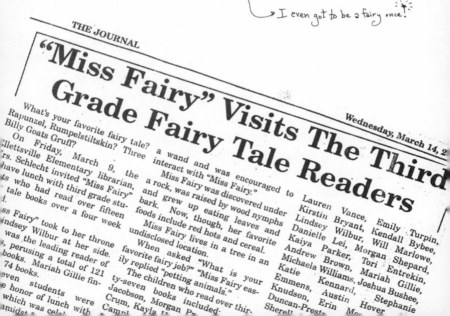

THE JOURNAL

"Miss Fairy" Visits The Third Grade Fairy Tale Readers

Wednesday, March 14, 2

What's your favorite fairy tale? Rapunzel, Rumpelstiltskin? Three Billy Goats Gruff?

On Friday, March 9, the Cllettsville Elementary librarian, rs. Schlecht invited "Miss Fairy" have lunch with third grade stuts who had read over fifteen tale books over a four week [...]

ss Fairy" took to her throne indsey Wilbur at her side. was the leading reader of 121 books, perusing a total of 121 74 books. Mariah Gillie fineven students were e honor of lunch with which was cel[...] amidst [...]

a wand and was encouraged to interact with "Miss Fairy." Miss Fairy was discovered under a rock, was raised by wood nymphs and grew up eating leaves and bark. Now, though, her favorite foods include red hots and cereal. Miss Fairy lives in a tree in an undisclosed location.

When asked "What is your favorite fairy job?" "Miss Fairy easily replied "petting animals."

The children who read over thirty-seven books included Jacobson, Morgan P. Crum, Kayla [...] Camp[...]

Lauren Vance, Emily Turpin, Kirstin Bryant, Kendall Bybee, Lindsey Wilbur, Will Marlowe, Danielle Lei, Morgan Shepard, Kaiya Parker, Tori Entrekin, Andrew Brown, Mariah Gillie, Michaela Williams, Joshua Bushee, Katie Emmens, Kennard, Knudson, Austin Hover Duncan-Preste, Erin Stephanie Sherell [...]

but I long for large chunks of uninterrupted time. The funny part is whenever I *do* have large chunks of uninterrupted time, I begin to feel confused and purposeless. Like everyone else has Somewhere to go, Something Important to do. And I don't have anything at all. When all my time belongs to me it doesn't seem quite as valuable anymore. I eat too much and sleep too much and watch all of those forensic-science documentaries on TV. That's why I try to be gainfully employed at least part of the time. And, like Edward Albee, I choose my work carefully. He said he was willing to work "any job so long as it had no future." (I'm going to remember that line for my next job interview!) He worked in an ad agency, sold books and records, and worked for Western Union for a while before he became a successful playwright.

Provided you are serious about your creative work, I recommend the shit job over the corporate job nearly every time. There's nothing wrong with selling sixty-four-ounce buckets of thirst-quenching soda at your local filling station while you try to get your band off the ground. True, you may have your family worried sick and things for you may be quite difficult at times, but you probably aren't going to starve to death. Some icky day jobs actually turn out to be pretty good.

When he was in the army, my friend Doug had the ultimate shit job—literally! Aside from digging holes, unloading trucks, and setting up and tearing down tents, he was occasionally tapped for "burning the shit" during Desert

Shield/Storm. To avoid the spread of disease in the encampment, it was necessary to incinerate everyone's poo in a fifty-five-gallon drum. Three parts diesel to one or two parts gasoline (Doug can't quite remember) had to be poured over the whole mess and set ablaze. He said it took four hours of intermittent stirring to powderize the poo, but the job wasn't nearly as bad as it might sound. For one thing, no one wanted to be around the flaming vat, so it had to be dragged some seventy-five yards away from everyone else. In between stirring, Doug could sit back, read a book, write a letter, rest. He told me, "I went into it thinking that I had hit bottom, but to my surprise it was like a refreshing visit to a spa." You never know.

But plenty of other jobs *are* indescribably horrible. My friend Benjamin made two dollars an hour working as a groundskeeper for a hospital back in the 1960s. He said, "The day I finally quit, it was a windy day, and it was Malathion day. They used to spray that all over the trees and bushes. . . . The stuff was blowing back on us, and I was quite relieved when I got the call to go down to the morgue.

"They needed me at the morgue lift. It was an amazingly hot, humid day. Apparently . . . a corpse had exploded. This caused the excrement that had been in the dead person to literally paint the walls of this morgue lift. It was quite thick, copious stuff. So I had to get down below this big scissor lift with—to his credit—the head of the groundskeeping crew, a gentleman by the name of Mr. Baggett. I think we just had cloth rags and our bare hands, and we were trying to scrub this tarlike substance off the walls. The stench just made your eyes roll back, it was so heady. And it was so powerful that this groundskeeping guy started coughing uncontrollably and, at some great seizure of a cough, his teeth went flying out, and they stuck into the wall in this corpse shit. I didn't even know he had false teeth until then. The whole scene of it there in the oppressive heat . . . the dreadful remains of somebody dead and this wheezing . . . and my boss . . . his teeth. I said, 'I need to go.' I laid low until three-thirty and got the hell out."

If you think your job is bad, it looks to me like things could always be worse.

And you're in very good company, too. Did you know that John Candy sold paper napkins door-to-door before he became an actor? That Steve Buscemi drove an ice cream truck? Jerry Seinfeld even sold lightbulbs over the telephone! In an interview with *GQ*'s Alan Richman, Seinfeld said it was a *tough job. There's not many people sitting home in the dark going, "I can't hold out much longer."* He also sold costume jewelry out of a little cart in front of Bloomingdale's.

Having the desire to "make it" is, of course, not enough. You have to have talent. In addition to working hard at their day jobs in order to sustain their dreams, these guys had real talent. You'll need that too.

Provided you have raw talent and plenty of moxie, the next time your folks ask you what you're going to do with your life, you can tell them about John and Steve and Jerry and all the hundreds more just like them. Better yet, tell them this: "Susan knows it's just a matter of time before I get somewhere with my creative work!" (Of course, then they'll say, "Who the hell is Susan?" and your house of cards will collapse . . . but I really do think you are on your way.)

SURVIVING CORPORATE CULTURE

I was Corporate Girl for a really long time—at least by my standards. As a commercial print broker for a newspaper, I made enough money to begin *The Lost Soul Companion* project, so that's good, but otherwise it was yucky.

A handful of people there were substantial and kind, but so many others were just well-dressed husks. You could almost tell how much money different people made by how loud and clicky their shoes were and how quickly they pounded around the building. I took to stealing earplugs from the pressmen in the back so I could block out the fat cats laughing just a little too loudly about Revenue Streams, "Buy-In," and Gantt Charts.

Not long after I got an _official_ book deal with Random House, I quit my steady job at the newspaper. When my editor at the publishing house found out, she seemed very concerned for me. I must've looked like some foolish hayseed from Indiana. You know, the kind with more fingers than teeth who buys a top-of-the-line Jeep Cherokee the minute her book advance check clears. But I didn't quit because of an influx of money. I left because I felt so tired at the end of every day that I could nearly lie down on the floor and die.

The Japanese have a saying: "The nail that sticks up will be hammered down." It is a kind of subtle threat to unconventional souls. To be successful one must not attract too much attention. One must behave appropriately and always follow The Rules, even if they don't actually make good sense. I believe most corporate environments operate on this principle.

(I'm sure I'll hear about this later, but I'm saying it anyway!)

Let's say you *do* land a corporate job—you even have your own cubicle and your family is so proud of you and now your mom can tell all her friends that her son is a "coordinator" at a software company. The pay may be better than what you'd get working as a janitor somewhere, but the hidden costs to you may be very high.

I remember so many Important Meetings I was forced to attend. They always started with a nonsensical agenda, complete with Roman numerals. People would talk and talk and I would strain to comprehend what they were talking about. For the longest time I thought I was just stupid, that everyone else understood the acronyms and the goofy business jargon just fine. ("Grossman can run an MBA and handle the general administrivities.") But then I got brave. I started asking what different things actually *meant*. I was stunned to discover that no one could ever really explain what was being discussed and that others in the meeting confided that they'd never understood what was going on either. When I realized that most of those meetings were a giant charade, I couldn't tolerate them anymore. (Wasting time like that is a sin!) I ducked out of them whenever I could. Sometimes I'd get trapped, though. Some meetings went on for an hour, hour and a half, and we'd still accomplish nothing. Invariably, my attention would wander to one young executive's strange hairdo, and I would have to grab the arms of my chair to keep myself from smooshing it down with my hands while she was in mid-sentence.

If you have any creative streak, you'd best hide it. If you have any common sense, don't be disappointed when you find out there won't be any need for it in your corporate job. If you strive for simplicity and seek elegant solutions to most problems, you won't be worth much to Management. As far as I can tell, cream doesn't rise in corporate America.

*Orbit the Hairball...

Many large companies do not value creativity, and some are downright hostile to Lost Soul types. If you are stuck in a very bad place, you might consider devouring Gordon MacKenzie's book *Orbiting the Giant Hairball,* an excellent corporate-survival guide for creative people. Mr. MacKenzie was a free spirit with such a magnetic personality that he was able to convince his company—Hallmark Cards—that he should create a new department called the Humor Workshop, and, in his final years with Hallmark, hold the position of "Creative Paradox."

I think some people are afraid of what they can't control or what they can't fully understand. MacKenzie says that the magical and unpredictable elements of creative genius are very threatening to society, which, in turn, *appoints its clandestine cartel to put a cap on imaginative brilliance.* He continues, *As old as civilization, the Genius Cartel is an originality-suppression agency that permeates our lives. It tyrannized Galileo into recanting the fruits of his own scientific genius. It handed Socrates a cup of hemlock, put a match to Joan of Arc, and fomented the crucifixion of Christ.*

Among its collaborators, the cartel numbers lawmakers, lawkeep-

ers, bureaucrats, clergy, teachers, parents, siblings, husbands, wives, lovers, co-workers, bosses, friends, acquaintances, and total strangers. Anyone who, having surrendered to this status quo, has become adverse to change.

Be a clam...

One way to survive your corporate job is to clam up like my friend Josh did. Management moved him into the cubicle next to mine, and I swear he didn't speak for at least a month and a half. When he finally did I learned that he plays the banjo and writes really good screenplays. He's a very private person, who showed up and did his job and, rather than get too involved jousting at corporate windmills, kept to himself. Of course, he goofed off as much as possible, too. Sometimes I'd catch him surfing the Internet, placing bids on obscure movie posters. Having Josh around made my workdays much more bearable. You might try finding a secret Josh of your own where you work. There has to be at least one around there somewhere.

Just scram...

Even with Josh around, I still wanted to leave. But I stayed and stayed. In part it was my giant ego that kept me there for too long. I was certain that the company would be Crushed by My Absence if I ever left and how could I do that to them? Ha! My seat was still warm when they found my replacement. . . .

When I was finally ready to leave my company, some people cautioned me against it. Your co-workers may do the same. They may ask: Is it really such a good idea to leave all of that security behind? I wonder if they have our best interests in mind or if they feel stuck and want us to be stuck too.

☆ Prodesse Quam Conspici

Not everyone has the option of just scramming, of course. Some people have families to support or piles of debt to attend to. New jobs aren't always easy to come by, and it can take a year or so before a new company will offer you benefits. If you *must* stay where you are but you don't know how you'll manage even another couple of months, there is hope.

At least that's what my brother says, and I'd listen to him, since he's quite well off (and I still think of fabric-softener sheets as a luxury item). Between us, I got the troubled, sensitive streak and Brother got most of the brains. Now he's a

→ I've called my brother "Brother" instead of his real name since I could talk...

77

mechanical engineer at a large corporation, and he has found a way to make things work.

I showed him a rough draft of this part of my book, and he really took me to task for being so limited in my view of corporate culture. This is what he told me: "Surviving in that environment and doing what you think is right and being creative is possible. It's a hard road. It takes a lot more effort than just shutting up or quitting, but I think it's worth-while."

Brother says there is a "corporate immune response to creativity," which must be quietly subverted. He explained, "In general, if you are a creative individual in a corporation, the people that you will struggle against are comfortable with certain processes . . . a certain way of doing things. As a creative contributor to the corporation, you represent change or a threat to the way things have been done. In order to effect change—to effect real change—you can't get it all at once. You can't rush in and meet the opposition headlong because you'll get beaten down. . . . So figuring out how to stage it . . . you basically sneak it in in bits and pieces and before long they look around and everything is changed, but it's the status quo now. They've sort of been silently, subversively brought along."

By bringing the others along with your own imperceptible influence, you work to make your position within the corporate culture satisfying. In the long run, maybe you'll even grow to enjoy your work since you can actively accomplish your own goals rather than blindly embarking on upper management's latest wild-goose chase.

He and his colleagues work by the Latin motto *Prodesse Quam Conspici,* which means to accomplish rather than to be conspicuous. It points to a quiet diligence and force of will that I admire. "*Prodesse Quam Conspici* means trying to achieve something without trying to be showy about it or grandstand. We took it a step further . . . not only are you trying to do things . . . trying to demonstrate your greatness through your works rather than through what you say, but you're trying to accomplish things in a way that is not conspicuous, that is in fact . . . almost insidious from the perspective of the corporate immune system," he said.

The way he achieved this was to know who his friends were and to know his enemies as well. He explained, "You need to know the people who are not receptive to change, and you need to react differently when you're dealing with them to not set those immune-system defenses on edge." Something else to remember: "The impediments to making those innovative leaps—a lot of the managers that you struggle against—are close to retirement. They're not going to be around forever."

Next Brother found a champion—someone with more sway who believed in his secret vision. "A better word is a patron. In corporate culture you can find someone to act as a patron who . . . will support what you're trying to do—within his ability," he said. "Your patron has to have more influence than you. He can be heard when you can't."

Just as important as finding a champion is making sure that your convictions are watertight. "If you've come up with a truly creative idea and it proves itself sound through study, that's hard to refute. At some point you can accrue an overwhelming body of evidence that will cause [your detractors] to wither," Brother said.

"It may also take extra time. This may be something you have to do on the sly—on your own time. It takes an extra commitment sometimes. That's why I say this is a hard road to go, because you may find yourself doing what the suits want and on the side doing what you think is right." That kind of double duty is a temporary sacrifice—one made with an eye toward a happier future. "Once you've got the story put together in a way that can't be refuted, then the real work that you were always about—your vision and goals—can bubble up to the surface and be the real thing that you work on," he explained.

Brother warns that this path takes a supreme force of will. It can be exhausting and miserable, and you and your colleagues must provide your own support system. Finally, what if you *do* succeed in subverting the system? "Let's say you're successful and this creative jewel that you've been nursing along becomes the status quo. Ultimately, if you're in a large company it passes beyond your ability to care for it and you have to let it go. It was your vision, but other people are going to do things with it, and it may not be what you had intended. You have to let it go. One of the things you've got to do at that point is . . . look for the next challenge."

If you *are* able to stick it out in corporate culture, you'll probably make a lot more money than I do. And money can give you entitlement to feed your creative passions. (But then there's the problem of finding the *time* to do what you really love. . . .)

TIME, MONEY, MUSHROOMS

You can think that you don't have enough time or money to do what is important to you, but, provided you're made of pretty strong stuff, there is an alternative to the regular day job. My friend Nate's a big believer in seasonal work—he lived in Kodiak, Alaska, for about seven years, working off and on as a fisherman—and it just may be the answer for artists wishing to buy themselves some time.

Nate's an adventurer/adrenaline junkie/ceramicist/metal sculptor/welder. (And, just so you know, his eyes look like melted chocolate.) He's also a sometimes painter/sometimes musician/sometimes photographer. He says *nothing* is something he wants to do all of the time. (That's not to say that he is someone always wishing to do *nothing;* rather, he is someone who seems to want to do lots and lots of *different* things instead of sticking to one or two for The Rest of Time.) As a result, seasonal work has been very good for him.

"Since I left college," he said, "mostly I'd been a fisherman, which leaves six months out of the year when you don't have to work. And so in between six months you could do whatever you want, play music in a bar for fifty dollars a week and free beer or travel, work weird jobs. I've kind of gotten into that habit of having six months to myself.

"There are a lot of artists that do that. Alaska's full of artists who are seasonal. It seems that an artist's energy level drops off in the winter. A lot of us suffer from [seasonal affective disorder]; that was part of my problem with having a steady job. Come January or February, I couldn't get out of bed. I just couldn't. Waking up at seven in the morning was just physically impossible."

Something equally impossible for Nate is putting off projects that are very important to him. His zeal got him fired once. "I got fired off a fishing boat," he said. "I spent a year straight out at sea. I was getting burned out. It was really hard work, long hours. I signed on for a salmon season; we were out in the middle of the ocean, and I had this project that I'd been wanting to do for the past six months. . . . [It was] a ceramic-tile fisherman's memorial for the city of Kodiak. It was six feet by four feet or something. It's around the flagpole at the center of town. I had sketches. I had it all worked out how I was going to do it, and I still had three months to go bouncing around the ocean. And my frustrations were revealed enough

82

around the crew that they finally decided to let me go. So then I got to do my project. So there are downfalls there."

 "Did you have enough saved up that you could do that?"

 "Yes. Fishing had its rewards financially. The project took me eight months from beginning to end. . . ."

 "So you were unemployed for eight months?"

 "Yeah. I was surfing a lot. . . ."

 "And you just lived on your savings from fishing?"

 "Right. At the time I wasn't rich. I had ten thousand dollars. The cost of living there was really high. It was over a thousand dollars a month for my house. . . . It was a nice year, but within the last two months of the project I was starving. I mean absolutely starving. I had four packages of ramen noodles left. It was bad."

After the project was done, Nate went back to fishing. He explained, "I didn't have enough money to eat. That's how I ended up becoming a captain. There weren't any jobs around, and there was an empty boat. I asked the guy if I could use it and he said yeah. So I went fishing. And, I remember, the first fish I caught I was so excited, not because I caught a fish but because I was hungry. Right away I cooked the fish and ate it. It was a strange, different kind of life."

Nate says he has a cycle. "I lived with a girl for a while in Alaska . . . and I was bitching about my cycle one day. You know, sometimes I'll have thirty thousand dollars and, six months later, I won't have anything. I spent it all on paintings or sculptures. . . . I buy art from other people or trade and sell. I'd spend it all and then I'd be down in the dumps and all depressed because I was broke.

"She said, 'I think you like your cycle.' I never thought of that. Maybe I do. Because I'm more creative when I have the need to be . . . when I'm frustrated or I'm broke.

"I used to drink a whole lot. My cure for that was every time I felt like going to the bar . . . instead I'd turn around and I'd grab a piece of steel and start cutting it. I'd try to occupy my mind; that's how I started doing art. Instead of going to the bar and spending fifty dollars, I'd spend fifty dollars on something to create. You go just as broke, but at least you've got something to look at in the end. It adds up after a while."

There are other well-paying seasonal jobs if you are particularly fearless or simply know where to look. "I scraped ice off houses. I got danger pay for that. The north sides of houses freeze up during the winter—two inches of ice," Nate explained. "I was the guy that got up there and busted the ice off. It was great but it was really dangerous. You're up three stories on a two-inch sheet of ice walking around. . . . The jobs that pay really well for short periods of time are really dangerous. And they don't last long."

Not all seasonal jobs are dangerous, though. "Last year I was out in the country, and I saw this flyer that said, PICK MUSHROOMS! This guy was paying two dollars a pound. I thought, Oh, that sounds interesting. Maybe I'll try that. They give you a picture and tell you where you might find them. It turns out I was really good at it. . . . I think I made two thousand dollars in two days picking mushrooms." I know it sounds crazy, but the giant mushrooms were perfectly legal. . . .

At least for now, Nate has hung up the seasonal work altogether. He has a "steady" day job at which he works forty to fifty hours a week, because his current artistic outlet—metal sculpture—is very expensive. I think he still longs for the open ocean, though. "The thing I miss most about being on the ocean is that's where I got all of my ideas. I'd sit out there for six months without any social stimulation. It's kind of like sitting in a jail cell—with the chance of sinking, of course. But you have plenty of time to think. You wake up in the morning and you see the sun, and you see the whales.

It's just beautiful, and it's very stimulating mentally," he said.

Nate has been at his steady job for almost a year now, and he says it's driving him nuts. "It sucks. It really does, because it drains so much of my energy. It's hard to loan your brain to someone for eight hours a day and expect to get it back in the same order, you know?"

He admits that the urge to just pick up and go is almost overwhelming. "I make future plans every day, but they change. Right now I have a real internal conflict. I don't know whether or not I have enough faith in art to stay. . . . I've been saving up for a while to buy new equipment, but maybe one day I'll go to the bank and say, 'That's enough money for me to go to Guatemala!' "

I suspect Nate will be back to his old ways again, sooner rather than later.

Seasonal work may sound far-fetched. Certainly, it's not what your parents might want for you, but if you don't have many attachments or obligations, and if you want time to do your own thing badly enough, you might be tempted to risk falling in love with the choppy seas, scaling tall buildings, or skulking around in the woods for impossibly large mushrooms.

LA, THE STARS, AND THE MOON

If you believe that you haven't gotten "anywhere" with your acting or music—your Passion, whatever it may be—because you live smack dab in Iowa, I say nonsense! Still, lots of Lost Souls flock to New York or Los Angeles because they are sure that opportunities abound and that Fantastic and Marvelous Things are in store for them.

For instance, I learned that my friend Shaun fully intends to move to LA in the fall. He *does* play a mean guitar, but he has no job lined up yet, nor any place to live. The timid three-quarters of me says he might as well go set himself aflame, but maybe things will work out better than that.

Shaun is dark-eyed and delightfully willful, so really there's no point in my telling him that his success doesn't have to depend on this move to a gigantic and faraway place. (Of course, maybe I am just projecting my fear of the unknown onto the adventurous lad. I am, after all, too afraid to drive in downtown Indianapolis.)

To shed a little light on this thing that I know so little about, I spoke to Tim Grimm, a musician and actor with plenty of big-city experience. You may have seen him in such films as *Clear and Present Danger, The Insider, Backdraft,* and *Mercury Rising.* (He has played lots of men in suits—security guards, FBI, CIA, reporters, the occasional priest.) He has acted in regular television series and in theater productions too, and he lived and worked in Los Angeles for six years. And then he did the unthinkable: He moved to the Midwest, where he and his wife—actress Jan Lucas—are raising a family.

"For the years that I was in Los Angeles," he said, "I was—on the surface, at least—comfortable. I certainly was working a lot and was successful in that vein and was doing well and making money . . . depending on how much merit we give that. But for me personally, it crept up on me . . . in a year or so—in the last year that I was out there—that there was more to life than what that place had to offer me."

Tim's idea of success is much different than that of many of his peers. "For a lot of people in the acting business, there's a strong desire to be 'recognizable.' . . . In my experience in LA, a lot of people really are out there to try to be a star. And you've got thousands and thousands of people out there, and that is their goal.

"My definition of success is living where I want to live and leading the lifestyle that I'm comfortable living, being in a place that I can very happily raise my family."

But the people he left behind in LA "don't quite get what I'm doing out here. . . . My unwillingness to spend big chunks of time out there hurts my chances [of getting more work in LA]. You've got to kind of keep your foot in the door. Almost at any level—I mean, maybe there are ten people in the world who are well known enough that they can be hermits and still get called [for acting jobs]. But beyond that, everybody else, you've got to still have your foot in the door and you've got to still put your face in front of them every now and again."

Still, Tim maintains that the extra effort is worth it. It's been two and a half years since he's been in LA, but he's still got plenty of acting work in Chicago on the stage and in television. Also, he receives residual payments from previous projects.

I've always thought that a person doesn't actually need to be in New York or LA to launch an acting career (or a career in any creative field, for that matter). Truly, it seems as if it can be done properly elsewhere. Tim said, "I think that talent really does eventually rise no matter where a person is. . . . It's, of course, trickier to make a living being an actor anywhere but one of the three major metropolitan areas in the United States, unless you're in a community that has a full-blown repertory company of which you're a member and [where] you've got a guaranteed amount of work per year."

Although there are fewer and fewer active repertory companies, Tim says there are still a few places worth considering. Ashland, Oregon, for instance, features the Oregon Shakespeare Festival, which houses a large number of actors and directors for at least a nine-month season. That could serve someone with an interest in acting on the stage, but what about acting on TV and in movies? It's got to be LA, right?

Nope. Tim said, "I would borrow a phrase that an acting teacher of mine—Philip Kerr—once told me: 'Don't go to LA unless you're invited.' " That's not to say you shouldn't *visit* LA once in a while to get your feet wet, but there's a better place for actors just starting out. Tim advised, "I encourage people—especially people who are just getting out of college—to head to Chicago. There are a lot more opportunities . . . especially if a person is looking at being—at least for the time being—a stage actor or actress. There are just so many companies coming and going and established companies that are open to new talent, and the media is very supportive of all of the theaters—Equity and non-Equity. It's vastly different from New York in that regard, in that a young company with not a lot of funding can put together some things literally in garage spaces or really funky spaces and the *Chicago Reader* will come and review it. And there's an audience for it." Chicago also does its share of television

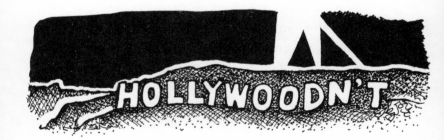

production, and film work comes through the Windy City from time to time as well.

Tim got his big break while he was based there. He'd been out of grad school just two years and had done a couple of shows at the Goodman Theater when his agent, also based in Chicago, helped him to secure work in LA for a CBS television pilot. He recalled, "They were trying to do a television version of *Steel Magnolias*. They had just a fantastic cast—Sally Kirkland, Elaine Stritch, Polly Bergen, and Cindy Williams—and I was the one male. It was quite a trip. I literally flew to LA, met with the director and producer, got the go-ahead, and the next day I was on a plane to Louisiana. I was down there for two weeks shooting this pilot. . . . That opened the doors in LA because, even though the show did not ultimately go, it was word on the street, so to speak. ('Gosh, who did they get to play the guy?') They had trouble—I laugh about this—they had trouble finding the right guy in LA. They've got tens of thousands of actors. . . . It was a mixture for me of luck, of being in the right place at the right time, and having a little bit of what they wanted."

Tim exudes a calm and simple satisfaction—partly, I think, because of his realistic goals and expectations. "I never wanted the moon. . . . I just wanted to do the work I enjoyed and make a living at it." Provided you're not expecting the moon, Tim says you *can* have it all—a creative career *and* a comfortable sense of place and home.

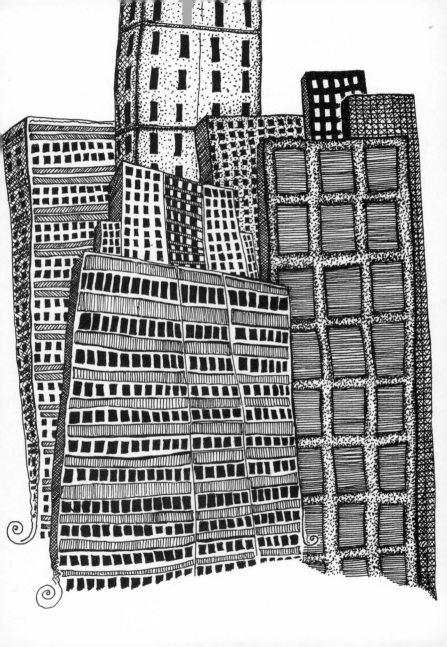

WHAT ABOUT NEW YORK?

When Ben Rinehart completed his MFA in printmaking from Louisiana State University, he looked around and thought, *What now?* He remembers, "I realized that, with my artwork, I had kind of tapped that area of the country out. . . . Artistically speaking, I really needed to rejuvenate myself, and I decided to move to New York." It wasn't always easy, but Ben is happy and making it in the Big Apple. In case you're hell-bent on going there too, here's how he's managed to get by so far.

Ben definitely hit the ground running. Although he did have a small nest egg and the luxury of staying on his sister's couch for a little while, he was on his feet with startling speed. "My focus in those first few months was, I need to find some sort of job so I can stay here. That was really all that was in my head. . . . I told myself that I wanted to stick with something that was at least somewhat related to the art world. I wasn't willing to give that up. I didn't want to go to any sort of temp agency and struggle along that way, and I wasn't interested in waiting tables."

Instead, he found an art-handling job—mounting, re-framing, repairing, and shipping artwork for a successful midtown gallery. "I was running my portfolio around for about a month and a half—probably at least four days a week. It was great because I got to know the city, but I noticed that you really need to be aggressive. Coming from the South, that was something that was a little bit foreign to me. You know, just keep putting myself out there." Besides his art-handling job, he occasionally taught classes and did birthday parties at the Children's Museum of the Arts.

"Moving from one state that is so completely [cheap to live in] to New York, which is so completely expensive, was a really big adjustment, and finding your worth as a human being, making sure that you're at least being paid enough that you can pay your bills, was very difficult," Ben said. Nevertheless, he was progressing. A cheap winter sublet in the East Village got him off his sister's couch.

Ben slowly worked his way into a regular teaching position, and more teaching opportunities cropped up based on the recommendations of new friends. Ben taught classes at the Center for Book Arts, the Friends Seminary, and the Children's Museum of the Arts.

When it was time to find his own place, Ben made two compromises. The first compromise was deciding to get a roommate, even though he didn't actually want one. And the other? "I bit the bullet and decided to move to Brooklyn," he explained. "That was one sacrifice that I was never willing to make when I first moved to New York. I thought, *I moved to New York, I need to stay in Manhattan proper, because that's what it means to move to New York.* Then reality set in. You know, Manhattan's really expensive!" As it turns out, he's very happy in what has turned out to be an artists' enclave.

Once he was fairly settled in New York, Ben was ready to take some new risks. "Since I do love teaching, I wanted to continue with that, but I also wanted to set up some sort of system for myself that would enable me to do my own work. . . . During that time it was very difficult for me to get my own artwork done. . . ." In order to make himself more marketable, Ben taught himself HTML, Photoshop, Illustrator, and Quark, and began freelancing as a Web and preprint designer. Now he was able to work fewer hours at his "day job" and free up time for his own creative work. (By the way, with his new skills, Ben put his portfolio on-line to save himself some legwork, and he wanted me to tell you this: The New York New Media Association (NYNMA) is great for people who want to do Web design. You can put a bid in for a listed job or you can put a posting up and let them contact you.)

Out of curiosity, I asked Ben, "What if a person moved to New York thinking he was only going to work as a fine artist?"

"You would probably get a lot of sad looks from people if you told them that," he answered. "It's a wonderful dream, but that's probably exactly what it is: a dream. I'm not saying that that's not something I don't want for myself, but I've realized that it's going to take some time to get there."

Someday Ben would like to support himself solely with his fine art, but he's not willing to sell out. "Some artists . . . will do a body of work based on the fact that they know that somebody will buy it. That's not why I do it. But I'm still very interested in making my artwork and . . . exhibiting my work. I'm just not necessarily married to the idea that I have to make fifteen thousand dollars off this show or else I'm screwed for the next six months.

"The thing that's kept me sane . . . is that I'm really just trying to get through my life and live a decent existence. I'm not trying to break the bank and fill my accounts up. . . . I'm doing all right for myself. . . . My idea of success is that, as an artist, you're happy with the work that you're producing, you're sharing it with people, and you're living a comfortable life. And for me it's not all about sports cars and mansions. I want to live somewhat of a normal life but be able to do my artwork and be passionate about it," he said.

Ben sounds content in the big city, and he thinks you can be too as long as you have what it takes. "My number-one advice for anybody that moves here—really that moves anywhere—and decides they really want to do something is that, one, they need to make sure they're passionate about what they're doing, but two, they need to have a drive."

I don't believe that you *have* to move to a big city to be a successful artist, but if it is your heart's desire, with a lot of hard work and perseverance, it can be done!

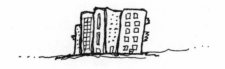

I'm glad Ben has done so well, but I suspect that New York City would kick me to the curb some five minutes after my arrival. I'll let the debate about success and geographic location rage on while I enjoy the obscurity of small-town life. Know this: Fellow cream puffs, there is hope. . . .

WHACK-A-MOLE ALTERNATIVES TO NEW YORK AND LA

I went to high school with a girl named Lora Emerson, who was a senior when I was a freshman, and I worked for her on the school newspaper. She and another girl were my editors. I remember they always smelled good and looked nice and they were very good at everything they ever tried, as far as I could tell. Usually around Christmas break one or both of them would come home from college and visit our newspaper staff.

I remember one of Lora's visits particularly well. I was now a senior, and soon I would be headed to Indiana University. Lora asked me if I knew where I was going to live yet. (Truly, I was so terrified of the whole prospect of leaving home that Mom and Dad had to force me to fill out my college application.) I told her coolly that I hadn't given it any thought at all—mostly because whenever I did consider my future I felt like I was going to throw up—but she didn't need to know that.

Anyway, she gave me some very, very useful advice about one on-campus dormitory. She said, "No matter what you do, don't live in Collins—that's where all the freaks live." Right then a door in my head opened just a crack, and I felt hopeful and calm. I knew I would live in this place.

As it turns out, many Collins residents were artistic souls—and some just looked artistic. They were pierced before piercing was popular. Some were spiky-haired, tattooed beauties. Atheists mixed with Jews for Jesus. Dreaded-up, ganja-smoking Rastas consorted with vampires. Best of all, no one minded if you were sort of like me either. I was home.

Now, if only Lora would come back and offer advice on the larger scale. Something along the lines of "No matter what you do, don't ever, ever move to Bisbee, Arizona. It's small and dusty and weird. . . ."

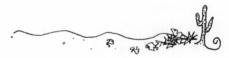

I happen to think that every Lost Soul deserves to live in a comfortable, colorful, and affordable community. Certainly, the very nature of the following undertaking will piss some people off, but I wanted to offer you a short list of decent alternatives to New York City and Los Angeles.

Of course, I know that by acknowledging these charming communities I put them at risk. Some critics might say, "Imagine the stampede of rubes, tourists, and sundry polluters!" And it's all my fault. Fortunately, I don't dare take any of this as seriously as all that.

And then there are the cities and small towns that I've left out. Well, it is a very short list, and I either left out locales because I never learned about them in the first place, or I left them out on purpose because—even though they may be artsy and cool—they have become altogether gentrified or are at least well on their way.

The most perfect place would be a creative, arts-supportive community with inexpensive housing, a reasonable cost of living, and plentiful jobs. To that end, I pored over really boring government statistics, spoke to some friends, and guessed a little bit to come up with my list of suggestions. As it turns out, this task was not unlike playing Whack-a-Mole.

Now in case you've never heard of Whack-a-Mole, imagine a pinball-style machine with a series of holes on its horizontal plane. Every so often, a mechanical bucktoothed mole pops out of one of the holes, and you have to smack him on the head to make him go back "underground." The object of the game is to smite as many of these popping-up moles as possible within a given time. As the game progresses, the moles begin to appear with increasing frequency. I've seen plenty of people play Whack-a-Mole and, believe me, the moles always win.

Anyway, while I was looking through my statistics, sometimes I hit the Artsy-Spot mole squarely and then, with grace and speed, whacked down the Affordable-Housing mole, only to be caught utterly off guard by the Terribly-High-Unemployment-Rate mole. It was virtually impossible to satisfy every category, but I sure did try. Finally, I owe it to you to say that I've never lived in any of these places, but you might consider them anyway.

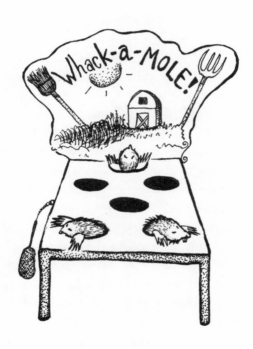

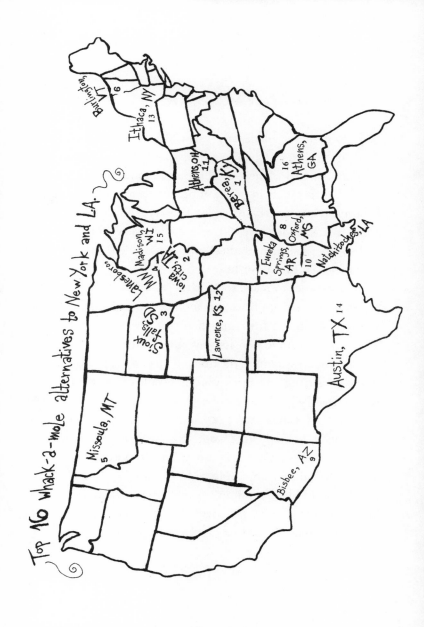

Top 16 whack-a-mole alternatives to New York and L.A.

Burlington, VT 6
Ithaca, NY 13
Athens, OH 11
Berea, KY 1
Athens, GA 16
Oxford, MS 8
Madison, WI 15
Iowa City, IA 2
Eureka Springs, AR 7
Natchitoches, LA 10
Lanesboro, MN 4
Sioux Falls, SD 3
Lawrence, KS 12
Missoula, MT 5
Austin, TX 14
Bisbee, AZ 9

TEENY PLANS, TINY PLANS, GIANT PLANS

Before I ever made any giant plans—starting my own publishing company and self-publishing a book count as giant—I had plenty of tiny plans. Some were even *teeny* plans. For instance, in hopes of becoming a published poet, I submitted my poetry to small literary journals and magazines at least twice a year. I won a few awards for my poems and was published sporadically in journals and small literary magazines you've never heard of.

And in order to make some extra cash, I once set out to sell my artwork—small prints, origami flowers, and marbled paper note cards—in one little gift shop that doesn't exist anymore. The shop was already on its way out and didn't have room to consign any new items at the time, so I had to go to Plan B. Plan B was me sitting on a brick wall by People's Park with my artwork attractively displayed nearby with a sign that read ARTIST AT WORK. ITEMS FOR SALE. I DON'T BITE. While passersby would stop to look, I quietly kept working on new pieces for art shows I did not yet have. On my best day, I made fourteen dollars and met my friend Benjamin. (He said "That's a great coat!" instead of hello, and I liked him immediately.) It was all on the up-and-up. I turned in my sales tax, I had a receipt book, and I was more than ready to use it. Nothing bad ever happened.

There is the occasional abandoned plan. The legal ramifications for my pornographic Muppet trading cards were much too horrifying, so I stopped after finishing just one card in the series—a full frontal nude of a naughty Kermit the Frog.

The things my *teeny,* tiny, and giant plans have all had in common: I considered each carefully, I tried my best to be realistic with my expectations, and, whether my idea was silly or not, I was still quite devoted.

Your goal can be small, and your plan doesn't have to be complicated, just very important to you. And it should be something you're serious about, because you may have to stick with it for a long time. The circus promoter P. T. Barnum advised, "Engage in one kind of business only, and stick to it faithfully until you succeed, or until you conclude to abandon it. A constant hammering on one nail will generally drive it home at last."

THE SUCCESS COMPANY

Marketing pro and author of *Guerrilla P.R.: How You Can Wage an Effective Publicity Campaign . . . Without Going Broke,* Michael Levine understands the power of a good plan: *We can't all be Beethoven, but we can all make music. . . . I'm not telling you to avoid dreaming big . . . but dreams occur while we're sleeping. I focus on the waking hours, when steel-eyed practicality goes a long way in making dreams come true.*

One thing that made writing and self-publishing my first book much easier was the fact that I had applied for a grant before I really got started. It must've taken me eighteen hours to answer all the questions on the application in just the right way. I waited and waited for a response. I checked my post-office box daily. Then the letter came: The Ella Lyman Cabot Trust regretted that they were unable to support my work at this time. Nevertheless, applying for the grant was time well spent, since I came away with a very detailed plan for what would become *The Lost Soul Companion* project.

$ $ $
Just because I didn't get a grant doesn't mean I'm against them. On the contrary, grants are quite valuable—even magical if you ask me. There are artists-in-residence programs, emergency living expense funds, and everything in between. There are grants for one-legged, blue-eyed speakers of Swahili. (Probably.)

If you don't think you're up to the task of applying for a grant, there are grant writing tutorial books and sites on the Internet to help you too. One of my favorite resources to look at in the library is Foundation Grants to Individuals.

$ $ $

As you probably know, not all plans are good, and sometimes it doesn't hurt to bounce an idea or two off a trusted mentor or friend before spending a lot of time and money on, say, populating Mars with a colony of Robotelope. (By the way, this is one of my friend Paul's advanced concepts. He says his robotic, antenna-antlered antelope would be patterned after "one of Nature's terrain-adapted designs." In the future, Robotelope could explore distant worlds, replacing their own battery packs through the use of "digit-enhanced little hooves.")

I know a guy named Rob who secretly started his own small, home-based business. None of his roommates even knew what he was up to until one of them noticed that the little card inside the back of their shared mailbox had been altered. All of their names were there—and a new name had been added in blue ink at the bottom: *The Success Company*. Now, with a name like The Success Company, you'd think business would've been great, but it didn't turn out that way.

Rob had a business phone line installed and placed some advertisements long before he'd even created his finished product—a booklet titled *Proven Dating Tactics*. It was to be a synthesis of other dating manuals he'd read, with added spins and twists of his own, but it was a long way from being completed. Besides, he'd encountered a problem he hadn't quite expected: Magazines and newspapers didn't want to accept advertisements for *Proven Dating Tactics* since it might be an unseemly product. He quickly rebounded from this setback.

"*How to Improve Your Chess Game in Ten Minutes*—or a half hour . . . I forget. It was just some of the key principles about chess that most people don't know if they're beginners. I placed that ad in *Discover* magazine, and I hadn't written [the chess booklet] yet. I was expecting to get maybe ten orders," he said. But he only got one or two—one from somebody in prison and one from some faraway country that he can't remember.

Rob was out a few hundred dollars and some of his time; certainly, things could've been worse. But they could've gone a lot better, too. Rob told me he wishes he'd done some things differently. "Rather than do what I did in the beginning, I think it's better to start out with something you enjoy and just do it because you enjoy it. And then if it turns into something, great. . . ."

Rob really likes the idea of being self-made. To that end, he started a new project—*Attracting Girls 101*—but he admits he hasn't touched it in years. "It's a challenge to work eight hours a day and then find the motivation to work another few hours on your own project, because it's still work," he explained. He remains hopeful though: "I'm confident that one of these days one of my projects is going to work out." With the right plan, it might.

MADAME PELE, BOLD PLANS, AND BAD LUCK

My mom was a latchkey kid back when it wasn't fashionable to be one. She wore her key on a long, red ribbon around her neck. Every day at lunchtime she would come home from school, cook tomato soup on the stove, and catch *Industry on Parade* on TV. Maybe that explains her self-sufficient nature and her hunger for success. Still, I think there's more to it than that.

Mom says that when Grandpa died, she felt like all of his dreamy, creative energy went out of him and flowed into her.

Because of her, I think most everything is possible. (She is herself a successful visual artist and art teacher.) But she's also taught me that some things just don't work out. The Discover Hawaii game was one of those things.

When Mom invented the board game Discover Hawaii, I was about nine years old. She and I would sit at the kitchen table and play her prototype over and over and over to work out the bugs before it went to press. I learned all about the scenic beauty, history, and people of the Hawaiian Islands. Over and over and over.

My prototype testing came in handy in the fifth grade. We were studying Hawaiian history and my teacher kept mispronouncing King Kamehameha's name. It was really starting to bother me so I raised my hand and said, "It's King Kah-may-hah-may-hah." I was just trying to help, but she completely ignored me and kept saying King KA-may-HA-may-HA instead. It sounded like someone was stepping on her chest every time she said it. Her tortured pronunciation made the Hawaiian unit much longer than it probably should've been. I guess sometimes it's best to keep your mouth shut. When I told Mom about it after school she just frowned and clucked her tongue.

She had produced one other game before this one, and it was a great success. She has a couple of other game prototypes too. But only one of Mom's projects is ominously referred to as "The Game." That's Discover Hawaii.

For years Mom couldn't even really talk about The Game without a box of tissues handy, but she was brave enough to discuss it here because she thought it might do Lost Souls everywhere some good.

Mom explained, "This was the only thing in my life that I ever tried that I couldn't make work."

When you think about everything that went wrong, you realize that this project was doomed from the start. Mom thinks some of it might've had to do with the fact that she took some lava home with her from a visit to Oahu.

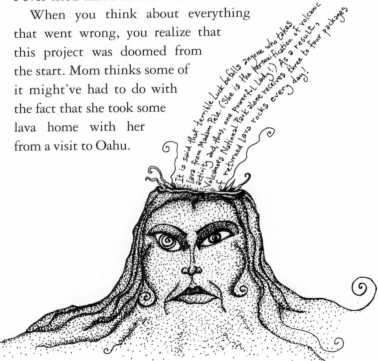

It is said that terrible luck befalls anyone who takes lava from Madam Pele. (She is the personification of volcanic activity and, thus, one powerful lady!) As a result, Volcanoes National Park alone receives three to four packages of returned lava rocks every day!

Nevertheless, when problems arose, Mom nearly always found ways to solve them. Since there really weren't any major printing companies in Hawaii, she had the games manufactured on the Mainland. Once they were printed, they'd have to be transported to Hawaii for sale—but how? Mom looked into using trains and boats with large cargo containers, but it really would've been best to ship her games by air. She knew she couldn't actually afford to have them shipped by air, so she implemented a rather Bold Plan.

A word about **BOLD PLANS**...

When you have ABSOLUTELY NOTHING to Lose, what's the harm in implementing the BOLD PLAN? What's the worst thing that can happen? Someone might tell you, "No." So? You've heard that before and it didn't kill you.

My mom took her hunk of cardboard to a boardroom full of United Airlines executives. She was the only woman there, and she had never done anything like that before. I think she believed so much in her project that she became extra brave and powerful at that moment!

"I went into this big room just like in the movies . . . with the big long table. All these men were sitting around the table,

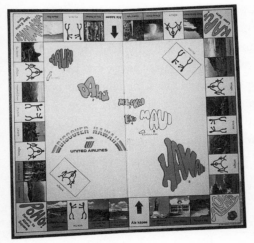

and there I was with my cardboard prototype. I told them that if they would fly the games for me from Indiana to Hawaii at no charge, I would be willing to put their logo on the board. And then I said, 'If you don't do it I'm going to Dallas next week to talk to American.' "

The executives said give us a few minutes and we'll talk about it. Then they said . . . Yes.

Still, some things Mom couldn't do anything about. "At the same time that I came out with the board game, electronic handheld games were the ticket and continued to be until Trivial Pursuit came along." Add to that the 1981 air controllers' strike plus distribution and marketing problems, and it was a real mess.

There was this strange thing called "Hawaiian time." People who lived in Hawaii didn't seem to be too constrained by watches, clocks, or deadlines. Mom explained it like this: "If they say they're coming to dinner at seven, they'll probably show up at eight. They're just so laid back; they're not like we are on the Mainland. When the Discover Hawaii games got over there, they put them into the warehouse and they didn't put them out on the shelves very quickly." Meanwhile, her loan at the bank was ticking away at twenty-one percent interest.

While we're on the subject of money, Mom mentioned that it is never, ever a good idea to use family money. Don't borrow from your mother, uncle, brother, sister, or anyone else you love dearly. Things might go wrong. Try to use OPM (Other People's Money) via venture capitalists, trusts, and foundations instead. If you can't find OPM, save up and use your *very own* money for your project.

Mom didn't make a business plan, but she wished she had. She also wishes she had started out smaller, and she regrets not checking out her printer and other vendors more carefully. She explained, "If I had just printed one thousand or two thousand games at first, I might have been okay. But the printer I worked with just raised the price per game so astronomically that I couldn't see any way to print a smaller quantity. I didn't understand the printing process. I didn't have a contract. The price just kept going up when we were in production." Whether you are choosing a recording studio for your first CD, a printer for your self-published book, or a talent agency to help jump-start an acting career, it is always a good idea to consider all of your options carefully. Ask for references and check them out!

Worse yet, Mom's lawyers were charging her one hundred dollars an hour for things she could've done for herself—like sending in her corporate minutes, for example. I really wish Mom's lawyers had been more honest with her. They could've quietly said, "You know, anyone can file these particular papers. You do that part on your own, and we'll help you with things you need a lawyer for." To their credit, maybe they thought Mom wanted everything done *for* her, but you can't meet her and actually still believe that.

If you're not sure if you need a lawyer for certain things, you might take a trip to your local library and do a little research. It is a little-known fact that reference librarians hold the Keys to the Universe.

There's also the Internet. Mom didn't have that luxury during the Discover Hawaii time, but it could've really helped. There are all kinds of helpful sites for inventors, musicians, actors, writers, artists, etc. (you can find a giant list of them at my Website, **www.lostsoulcompanion.com**).

Finally, it doesn't hurt to find a mentor of some sort. Talk to someone who's been around longer than you have, someone who's finished a major project or two of his own, someone who would like to see you succeed and believes in you and your project. Most communities have business incubators that may or may not be helpful, but you won't know 'til you try.

Hey, aren't business-y people stuffy and uptight? Some are.
But some aren't! It takes real creativity to be able to find a need and fill it. And it takes guts to create something from nothing and convince other people to spend their money on your goods and services. So the business-y people who haven't forgotten what it was like when they were just starting out their own massage therapy shops or art galleries or Internet service providers may just have some really good advice for _you_.

The most important things Mom took away from the Discover Hawaii debacle? Marketing and distribution can be even more important than the quality of your product. "Sometimes there are just too many variables, and you just can't control everything. But you have to control everything that you can."

The Tangled Black Scribbles & Other Pitfalls

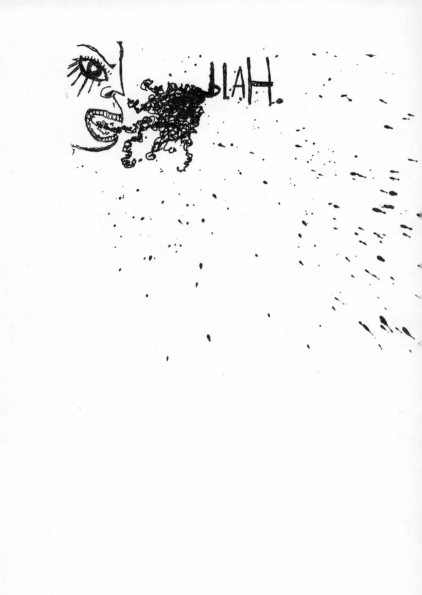

MEAN-HEADS, NICE-HEADS, AND WHEN TO KEEP QUIET

This may seem obvious, but Lost Souls (and Not-So-Lost Souls too) are wise to avoid really negative people. The extra discouraging ones barf up black scribbles instead of plain old words in conversation. After listening to them long enough, you can get all tangled up. You might even consider giving up on your dreams altogether. These Mean-heads will say things like "Why do you keep on writing those stupid novels? No one's ever going to read them anyway." Not to mention that the negative energy they give off is pretty contagious. Find Nice-heads instead and bask in their glow.

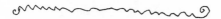

Sometimes it's not a matter of *whom* you talk to but *when* you talk to them. I get so hungry for feedback sometimes that I have trouble resisting the urge to show off my works in progress. Once in a while I'm actually delighted with something I've written, and I want to show it to the mailman and my roommate and anyone else who will look. This is sort of to elicit the same feeling I got as a kid when my mom selected my best drawings for exhibition on the refrigerator door. (Only this time it's like I've got Mom at gunpoint and I'm forcing things a bit.) Invariably, though, I am disappointed by the reactions I get. And then I begin to doubt myself. Especially in the early stages of a creative project, if I hear even one noncommittal "It's not bad," it can be enough to make me put it away forever.

I try to remember the words of Epictetus at times like these. He wrote: *Take care not to casually discuss matters that are of great importance to you with people who are not important to you. Your affairs will become drained of preciousness. You undercut your own purposes when you do this. . . .*

Other people feast like vultures on our ideas. They take it upon themselves to blithely interpret, judge, and twist what matters most to you, and your heart sinks. Let your ideas and plans incubate before you parade them in front of the naysayers and trivializers.

Most people only know how to respond to an idea by pouncing on its shortfalls rather than identifying its potential merits. Practice self-containment so that your enthusiasm won't be frittered away.

ABOUT AGENTS AND ONE WAY TO GET YOUR OWN

There are some people out there who can be trusted to offer you guidance and help when it's time. They are good editors, managers, publicists, colleagues, mentors, and agents, and they can be invaluable if you have access to them.

I think, of all of them, a good *agent* can make the most happen for you.

In my case, you probably wouldn't be reading these lines if it weren't for the fact that a literary agent agreed to help me look for a publisher.

Lots of people have trouble finding an agent, and I didn't actually think I'd succeed. Here's exactly what I did to find mine. First, I looked for books that were similar to mine in subject as well as flavor (*Inspiration Sandwich* by SARK). Then I looked at the acknowledgments pages of some of her other titles to see if SARK had recognized her agent there. She had. I figured that if the agent supported someone like SARK, then she might want to help me too. I searched the Internet and various literary trade magazines until I found the right address. I sent her a copy of my self-published book and a heartfelt letter. I'd determined that she was the best-suited agent for me and my project, and if she wasn't interested, my search would end there. Some things just aren't meant to be after all.

If you are casting about for an agent—whether literary or miscellaneous talent—I think doing your homework is a better use of time than just peppering every agent alive with requests for representation. Finding a reputable agent still doesn't mean easy street, though. . . .

"OH, GOD . . . WHY WON'T JUST ONE CITY EMBRACE ME?"

I am embarrassed to admit it, but I actually uttered these words aloud in my kitchen. My friend Paul was standing nearby when the ridiculous question tumbled out of my mouth, and he still giggles about it.

I tried to explain that I wasn't quite as arrogant as I sounded. After all, I wasn't asking for New York or Los Angeles. No, I told him, Wichita would be acceptable. Or Flint, Michigan, even. Wouldn't it be nice, I reasoned, to be able to say that *The Lost Soul Companion* was wildly popular in, say, Walla Walla, Washington?

Nevertheless, Paul suggested that perhaps it was unrealistic for me to expect an *entire metropolitan area* to "embrace" me. Perhaps. (What would it feel like to be "embraced" by an entire metropolis anyway? . . .) But I had been working so hard at getting the word out about my project, and I just wanted some tangible results. It happens that executing a vigorous marketing and publicity campaign *is* very hard work. It's also a test of endurance—kind of like college.

I have yet to meet an artsy-type person who actually enjoys the business side of his creative field. For better or worse, arranging media coverage and public events is usually part of your job if you are a self-published writer, a visual artist, part of a local circus troupe, or an up-and-coming Kenny G. Unless you have the money to hire a private marketing and public-relations firm to help (and tell me, what artist does?), you probably already know you'll have to spend a lot of your time and energy furthering your own cause.

Don't say I didn't warn you. Promotions work can be daunting enough to make most sane people lament dramatically in their kitchens. But it can be a lot of fun, too.

THE NITTY-GRITTY

I used to work at an arts and entertainment magazine where I had the opportunity to scrutinize all sorts of press kits. We received professional CD release packages from 4AD and Rounder Records pretty regularly. We also got press kits from regional visual artists and the occasional advance review copy of a new book.

I can tell you that the most professional-looking presentations got our attention ninety-nine percent of the time, and if they included graphics we could use, we were even more likely to give them the press coverage they sought. Lame-o press kits were the ones that arrived way too late for us to do anything with. Either that or they were full of misspelled words, grammatical mistakes, and too much confusing information.

> * Always try to send graphics with your press releases. If you need to, call ahead and see what format is acceptable for each publication you contact. Talk to someone in the production/art department long before you try to speak with the editor or reporter. A very established publication may also have graphic submissions guidelines on its website. If they specify black and white, glossy photos only, don't send them color slides (unless you __want__ to irritate them).
>
> *If you don't have a super-deluxe camera, that's OK. You can buy pretty decent, disposable 35mm cameras. And maybe you can ask a friend who's a good photographer to assist you. Maybe he'd even let you borrow __his__ equipment. You could clean out his bathtub in exchange...

As a result, I knew that the press kit I prepared to announce the release of my self-published book had to arrive in plenty of time, make sense, and look professional. I figured that bigger newspapers, magazines, and review journals probably don't even open their mail unless it looks interesting, so I used glassine (see-through!) envelopes for my press kit. That way my recipients would sort of have X-ray vision—enabling them to sneak a peek at the contents and, thus, become desperate to rip open the envelope. I included an advance review copy of my book, a well-written, short press release, a glossy black and white promotional photograph, and a toy compass.

100 toy compasses cost me $126. I illustrated the compass face, had color copies made, and then Mom and Dad and I assembled them by hand at the kitchen table. It sounds tedious, but it was fun. Promotional items can be attention getting, and I figure every little bit helps!

If you want to be really creative with your press kit, you might consider adding a small promotional item. Most towns have shops that sell business incentive items in case you're curious.

In addition to a good press kit, good timing is everything. Aim for a "slow news day" so you don't have to compete with the Monroe County Fair Queen contest. (In the event that you do receive some degree of media coverage, make my mom proud and be sure to send a nice thank-you note.)

As well as securing print interviews, I was able to set up some book signings and speaking engagements. At those events I made new friends and contacts, which invariably led to new opportunities for me and my project. For instance, after I contacted my local Barnes & Noble about a possible book signing, the manager there helped me contact the national office in New York to discuss widespread distribution of my book in other Barnes & Noble stores.

Sending out promotional postcards now and then was also a big help. I've heard that some actors hoping to land auditions even send picture postcards of themselves to casting directors. (By the way, one of the best printing resources I've found for this is a company called Modern Postcard. See the appendix for details.)

Despite my progress, there are plenty of things I wished I'd done differently with my marketing efforts.

For one thing, it didn't occur to me until it was largely too late that I should've pursued more television, Internet, and radio interviews. (They actually seemed easier to secure than print interviews, but more on that in "The Obnoxious Part.") In particular, radio is a good way to go—unless, perhaps, you're a visual artist. You can do radio interviews from home. You can do them completely naked if you like. No one needs to know.

Local cable-access television is also a very good untapped resource. Since not every town has a Tom Green to flood local channels with delightfully goofy content, there is still plenty of bandwidth to go around. I wish I had taken better advantage of that. But, like my friend Scott always said, "If wishes were horses, then beggars would ride."

The Obnoxious Part and the Magic Word

My worst marketing mistake of all: Sometimes I was a little overzealous—but it was only because my project is so important to me! This may just be my imagination, but I think I've been completely banned from the pages of at least one local publication because I was *Obnoxious.*

My shame is even greater because I should've known better than to pester the editor of a print publication. After all, I had myself been annoyed countless times by publicity seekers during my stint at the arts-and-entertainment magazine. But pester I did.

I should've listened to Michael Levine. *In Guerrilla P.R.: How You Can Wage an Effective Publicity Campaign . . . Without Going Broke*—a good book, by the way—he had this to say about newspaper reporters: *Avoid the hard sell. Saying "You have to cover this" just won't work. My reporter friends uniformly claim their disdain for pressure from outsiders. You must be willing to bend, even to the point of losing. Better to miss out this time and keep a friendly contact, rather than go for broke in an obnoxious manner and lose out permanently.* I went for broke.

In addition to my standard press kit, I sent the editor quite a few e-mail messages, "popped in" unexpectedly once or twice, and—the kiss of death—left about three hundred too many voice mails. Levine writes, *If the person you're trying to reach isn't in, don't always leave a message when you call. Sometimes media people rely on their voice mail to screen calls. If you leave two dozen messages, you will probably never hear from the reporter. Call with the intention of speaking to someone, but leave only a tiny handful of messages.* Oh, Mr. Levine, I knew better!

About tiny handfuls of things...
they seem special compared to great big barrels of things, don't they?...
I've heard that it's possible to be a little _too_ accessible. I know of one artist whose philosophy is: If you are a Mystery, people will be curious about you. If everyone — including the local media — sees you buying light bulbs at the hardware store, you could begin to seem very "normal" and, for an artist hoping to separate himself from the humdrum realm, that could be bad.

I'm sure you'll be able to finesse the print media better than I can. And once you feel comfortable enough, try contacting newswires and news syndicates too. They're always trolling for a good story, and they might be interested in your project.

There's one more thing too. The magic word. I was able to use it most successfully with everyone—except that one beaten-down editor. The magic word is: *confirm*. As in, "Hi, Mr. Biggles, I was just calling to *confirm* that you received my press kit." People like to be able to say yes. So if the

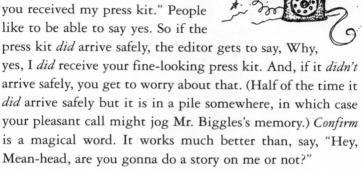

press kit *did* arrive safely, the editor gets to say, Why, yes, I *did* receive your fine-looking press kit. And, if it *didn't* arrive safely, you get to worry about that. (Half of the time it *did* arrive safely but it is in a pile somewhere, in which case your pleasant call might jog Mr. Biggles's memory.) *Confirm* is a magical word. It works much better than, say, "Hey, Mean-head, are you gonna do a story on me or not?"

Courting the media is a delicate matter. Magic words help. Carrying yourself professionally is advantageous. So is writing effectively and having clean hair. (Mostly just try not to be obnoxious like me, and you should be okay.)

JUMPING OFF THE BROOKLYN BRIDGE TO GET ATTENTION IS NOT A GOOD IDEA

Some people worship at the altar of the Publicity Stunt. I am not one of those people. Employ the publicity stunt if you wish, but, for the love of everything you hold dear, don't get carried away. Publicity stunts are often more trouble than they're worth. Just ask Dan Cameron Rodill.

The August 30, 1977 *New York Times* reported: *In an ap-*

parent publicity stunt for his latest literary effort, an aspiring playwright clad in a wet suit and flotation gear placed his unpublished manuscript on a railing of the Brooklyn Bridge yesterday afternoon and plunged one hundred and thirty feet into the East River. Police discovered a statement entitled "Playwright on the Bridge" in the unconscious playwright's wetsuit. According to reports, Rodill made the jump to draw attention to his play *The Dry Season* and *to make a statement about Indochina, unemployment in corporate-commercial society, the plight of New York and writers who would rather fight than quit.* Maybe he was just ahead of his time?

According to his roommate, Rodill had tried for months to market his latest play: *"He sent it out to places here and in Europe but nothing came of it."* That's when he decided to make a splash.

Although he'd planned and prepared for the stunt well in advance, he ended up with sundry internal injuries, including thirteen broken ribs and punctured lungs. He was hospitalized in critical condition for nearly a month. Adding insult to his injuries, *The New York Times* refers to him again and again as a "frustrated writer of unproduced plays" when following up on his medical condition. Surely this isn't the kind of attention he'd hoped to get. (Even now I'm a little squeamish about dredging all this up.)

By September 25, *not even the most obscure Off Off Broadway impresario had asked to see the script of the play* The Dry Season, according to the *Times*. Eventually, though, someone in

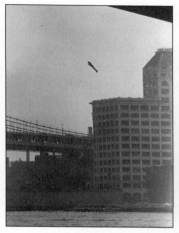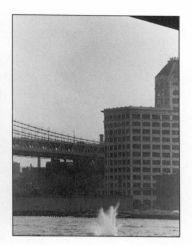

Paul Hosefros/NYT Pictures

Philadelphia *did* offer to produce his play, but I don't know how it turned out.

From what I can tell, Mr. Rodill already had a good career as a freelance journalist—by the time he decided to jump off the bridge, he'd already written pieces for *Newsweek,* the *Chicago Sun-Times,* and British and Japanese television stations—but maybe that didn't satisfy him.

I had hoped to speak to him about all this. I wanted to know if there was anything he wished he'd done differently and if his play was finally produced to his satisfaction. It seems, though, that he keeps a lower profile these days. As far as I know, he just wants to be left alone, and I certainly can't blame him for that. (I suspect that some publicity stunts' effects last long after one's bones have healed.)

In my own quest for publicity, I have been nearly frustrated enough to jump off something. Sometimes, no matter what you try, it still seems like you're invisible. Working within the You're Nobody in Your Own Backyard Theory, since Mr. Rodill lived in New York City, he might have had more success had he jumped from the San Francisco Bay Bridge instead. (But I certainly wouldn't want him to test that idea. . . .)

You're Nobody in Your Own Backyard

It's even in the Bible. Something about being a prophet in your own hometown. (As I am something of a heathen, I'm not good with biblical references.) I say it like this: You're nobody in your own backyard. For whatever reason, lots of creative people have a very hard time getting attention in their own towns. Artists can't always get local galleries to offer exhibit space. Local bands can't get gigs—or, if they *do* get a gig, no one shows up to hear them. Media coverage is almost nonexistent. It's especially bad in small towns. No, it's not just you.

I've thought about what could help make local artists more appealing. The answer is simple. Those "local" artists just have to be from someplace else.

Small towns like mine *love* covering artists and acts from

Louisville or Indianapolis or, ooh, Chicago. They have more cachet than anyone local ever could.

So one thing you can do to be "somebody" instead of "nobody" is to create, exhibit, or perform in other communities instead of the one you're in. Overseas experience is especially glamorous—even if it's just a tiny art exhibit in a coffeehouse in Brussels. But you can travel one hundred miles or so in any direction and try your luck just the same. You'll probably seem exotic. After quite a lot of this, you'll have honed your skills, acquired some valuable experience—maybe even some press clips—and your own town might decide you're not so bad after all. Notice I said *might*. I think you *can* win your town over, but you may have to win over the rest of the free world first.

WRITING, REJECTION, AND THE MACHINE

My friend Jeff has completed about two dozen writing projects, including short stories, novels, and children's fiction. For more than a year, one of his novels has been represented by a literary agent, but Jeff isn't consumed with thoughts of the novel being published. He says that would be like waiting for Christmas to come every single day. He explained, "It doesn't work that way. Editors and agents work on a different time schedule than everybody else does. The best thing that I've been able to do is to submit something to an agent and to an editor and then forget about it."

Jeff recommends that artists of all kinds—and writers in particular—accept this certainty: Once you've created something and sent it out, it's no longer entirely yours. It's only yours when you're working on it. There's no accounting for others' interpretations of your work. They may consider your project with an entirely different frame of mind. And, he says, since outside perceptions of your work are completely out of your control, the best thing to do next is to go on to a new project and not give the old one another thought. (That seems hard to me!)

It also doesn't hurt to prepare for rejection . . . just in case. Jeff's gotten two or three hundred rejection slips from agents and publishing houses so far. He plans to wallpaper his bathroom with them someday. Jeff thinks that a writer has to be a little bit of a masochist. He puts it like this: "[A writer] sends out a piece of [his] spirit and knows that it's going to be completely torn apart—or worse, ignored." He's rarely had someone say anything negative. Instead, "It's either been accepted or ninety-nine percent of the time has been completely rejected out of hand. It's been in a slush pile somewhere . . .

→ Jeff's EXASPERATED RANT

. . . and now some editorial assistant (you know Elaine from Seinfeld? This is one of her assistants) who's making eight dollars an hour and hates her job and is being beaten up by her boss is going through the pile. Even if a fantastic book were in this pile, no one is going to see it because this editorial assistant who probably just

graduated from Vassar is going through this pile, saying, "No. No. No. No." and sending it back with just this little slip of paper. (The things they send out have been photocopied fifty thousand times.)

Jeff continued, *I believe that most manuscripts come back unread. There's no way that a small staff with a couple of editors and maybe a dozen editorial assistants can read the kind of work that comes in—really give it a decent look through. Not just "Does this first sentence grab me? No. Okay." I think a lot of editors, if they got something that wasn't as polished as it could be, could work with the writer and come up with something really terrific.*

That sounds nice, but that doesn't seem to be the way things work. Instead, Jeff says, there is the great Machine to consider. "Very few people make money by writing, acting, painting, doing creative work. It may not have anything to do with the fact that you are a good writer or a good artist— or a bad writer or a bad artist. What you have may not be what the Machine wants right now.

"With writing, if one story that's very different from everything else comes along and it becomes the hot thing, then everybody wants that. There's no set of guidelines. You can send the same story to the same person five different times and it may meet their criteria one week and it won't the other weeks. There's no consistency and there's no logic to it. [Publishers] are trying to forecast public opinion and what will sell. They want Stephen King. They want *Bridges of Madison County*. They want these huge books. But they're not going to find this kind of blockbuster all the time, and they're going to turn down a lot of really good books."

That's why, according to Jeff, you shouldn't take those form rejection letters too personally. They may be hard to deal with, but as Jeff always says, "If you can't paper your walls with them, then you're not trying hard enough."

Rejections aren't all bad. Here's a really nice one that I got from *The New Yorker* about a year after I sent them a review copy of *The Lost Soul Companion*.

While we wish you every success with The Lost Soul Companion, and applaud your venture, it is unfortunately unlikely that we will be able to feature it in our pages.

The Editors

I have it hanging up on my wall most of the time, because it reminds me that my work must've struck a chord with someone in a pretty high place. Why else would they take the time to handwrite a rather kind response?

I also heard from the librarian at *Newsweek* magazine. He said that he doubted anyone in editorial would do anything with my book, but that he read it and really enjoyed it. So technically it's yet another rejection, but, again, someone was moved enough to respond to me. Those are the kinds of rejections that make being rejected not so painful.

WHAT TO DO WHEN YOU FIND YOUR ART HANGING IN A USED-FURNITURE STORE

Any time you put your creative work "out there" you are taking some risks. Rejection, disappointment, and public humiliation are all possibilities to consider when you offer your creative talents for public consumption.

For instance, musicians playing out in public hope that some people will actually show up to hear them play. They hope that the people who actually *do* show up won't boo them off the stage or pelt them with lit cigarettes. They hope that, maybe, there are reviewers in the audience and, if there *are* any reviewers in the audience, that they will be charitable. Finally, if all goes well, maybe they won't find their CDs—the ones they worked so hard to release—three at a time in the used bins.

The same goes for actors. Consider the story of poor Geoffrey Steyne, an actor back in the 1920s. Peter Hay explains in *Theatrical Anecdotes: As a play reviewer Heywood Broun was usually gentle, but one actor's performance so displeased him that he was moved to classify the young man, Geoffrey Steyne, as the worst actor on the American stage. Steyne sued, but the case was dismissed. The next time Broun reviewed a play in which Steyne appeared, he made no mention of the actor until the last sentence, which read, "Mr. Steyne's performance was not up to its usual standard."*

As for writers and artists, feedback is less immediate—but no less potentially devastating. Kind of makes you want to go back to bed, doesn't it?

Don't feel bad. It happens to everyone sometime or other. It's certainly happened to me.

One day a co-worker of mine said, "Hey, I saw your art for sale somewhere the other day." I didn't have any exhibits up at the time, so I couldn't imagine what he was talking about. He must be mistaken. But, no, he described "Puckitt Wins Bingo" perfectly, and, he added, it was just five bucks at Long's Landing Used Furniture. I pretended to be unfazed—even pleased—at the thought of my art hanging up in "Indiana's largest used-furniture store—in the big red barn just off Highway 46 East." But, truthfully, I was horrified.

I immediately thought it meant that *everyone* hated my work. That I was a failure as an artist and that I should just quit trying and go get a decent job.

I decided to visit my art. I wanted to be certain it was really there, and I needed to assess the situation for myself. There it

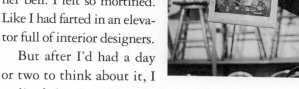

was, hanging in the very back—in the dining-room tables-and-chairs section— next to a quaint, rustic dinner bell. I felt so mortified. Like I had farted in an elevator full of interior designers.

But after I'd had a day or two to think about it, I realized that I could really be certain of only one thing: that *someone* had decided that this particular piece just wasn't worth keeping anymore. *Someone* isn't Everyone. *Someone* is just Someone. I guessed I could live with that.

Also, the fact that they brought it to the shop at all suggests that they thought *Someone Else* would find value in it. (Either that or they were just really desperate for some cash and thought they'd try their luck with all the cheesy crap they had in the closet.)

I'll never know for sure, and I'd probably go crazy trying to figure it all out anyway. It's just not worth getting too upset about because it was bound to happen sooner or later.

I know I'm not the first or the only creative soul that got a bit dented—maybe even temporarily crushed—in the line of duty. There have been so many others and there will be many more. If you find yourself among them, please remem-

ber me and the big red barn and know that you are in es-
teemed company. (an interesting aside that has little relevance
to the rest of this book...)

I used to work at Long's Landing Used Furniture. It was
my first job out of college. My folks had been pressuring me
to get a job, but they hadn't specified that they wanted me
to get a "real" job in the "real world." Of course, I knew that
they'd like to see me working in a law office or as a publicist
or something, but I decided to put my newly acquired English degree to work selling furniture instead.

Not long after I started, J.D., the store owner, put me in
charge of the mice. There had been a scene earlier, you see.

Claudia, J.D.'s wife, had put a glue trap out a night or
two before, and a tiny mouse had gotten stuck in it and had
been there for a very long time. Half of him was normal-
mouse and the other half was sick-gluey-panting-mouse. I
stuck it right in her face even though I knew she was terrified of mice, which I know wasn't very nice of me but I felt
righteous and indignant. To end the creature's suffering, I
took the glue trap with the half-and-half mouse outside the
store and brained him with a large chunk of cement by the
Dumpster. After that, J.D. put me in charge of the mice.
There would be no more glue traps. Instead, I used a large
metal trash can and great globs of peanut butter, like
this . . .

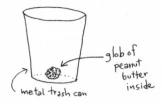

glob of peanut butter inside

metal trash can

. . . and every morning the trash can would be filled with three or four happy, well-fed mice. I would dump them out in the woods and catch them all again the next day. (I would've liked to put spots of fluorescent paint on their tails so that I could keep track of them, but I was, after all, being paid to sell furniture and not track the local mouse population.)

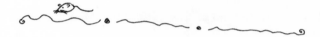

I was also supposed to fill the Coke machine and clean the bathroom. I used to hate refilling the Coke machine, by the way—until the secret fortunes, that is. I would write them on tiny strips of paper and then tape them to random cans of soda.

Any time customers would buy sodas, I would get all excited and watch as they put their money in, made their selections, and grabbed their cans out of the dispensing trough. Would they notice anything unusual? Maybe I made them too

Someone loves you terribly.

Soon you will swallow a cool and tasty beverage.

Everything will be all right.

beware. your neighbor is jealous of your car.

small. As far as I know, no one ever noticed the fortunes. But at least I knew they were there.

⟨ꙮ〜〜〜 • 〜〜〜 • 〜〜〜 ꙮ⟩

(See? I told you this had little relevance
to the book. Of course sometimes it's good to take
a break from what you were doing!)

HOPE FOR THE BEST . . . PREPARE FOR THE WORST

When you are ready to make your work public, it doesn't hurt to mentally prepare for all the possibilities. Here is the worst print review I've ever gotten:

ART
By Lydia B. Finkelstein

Five at Waldron

Back in Bloomington, at the Waldron Arts Center, five artists are currently exhibiting recent work. Susan Brackney's mixed media works of various personality types may, or may not, be funny depending on your sense of humor.

Paul Houseman, Kevin Titzer, and Thomas Zeta all work in three-dimensional forms with wood, combined with tin, clay, glass and other common materials. The three sculptors, all with connections to the University of Southern Indiana, also seem to be on the same wave length in their use of rather simple forms, but enhanced with painted tints and and surface treatments that change them into suggestive shapes that echo houses, shelters, birds, and secret hiding places.

The four really should have been installed alone because the effect of Brackney's very different and satirical images intrude on this community of inanimate presences that seem to have alighted in the Miller Gallery from some strange planet. The humor is muted and gentle.

I don't think she liked my stuff. Then again, since she couldn't seem to decide how many artists were exhibiting, maybe I should be glad that she at least mentioned me.

My friend J.J. used to be the music reviewer for our local newspaper. He once admitted to me that he always tried to find *something* nice to say in a review even if the rest of his column was negative. There were three reasons for this. One, J.J. is a very nice guy. Two, J.J. is himself a musician and relates to the artistic cause. (He once explained, "If I put at least one good sentence in, the band can pull that and use it in their press kit.") And, three, we live in a very small town in which reviewers can't afford to be brutal.

When J.J. couldn't find *anything* nice to say, he would just hem and haw and try to avoid reviewing the musicians in question at all. (So if you live in a small town and can't get anyone around to review you, that could be a bad sign—or it could just be a classic case of You're Nobody in Your Own Backyard.) If you live in a big city, brace yourself. Since critics are more insulated from crazy, temperamental artists like us, they can say pretty much whatever they want.

For centuries, many artists have viewed critics as inept and terribly spiteful at the same time. It has been said that a critic is "a legless man who teaches running." Coleridge called critics *Disinterested thieves of our good name: Cool, sober murderers of their neighbors' fame.* The last time I had Chinese food, my fortune cookie even had an opinion. . . .

Feeling a bit critical myself, I wonder, is that even a fortune and do I really believe that? Some philosophers choose the beleaguered critics' side. In *Human, All Too Human,* Nietzsche writes, *Insects sting, not in malice, but because they want to live. It is the same with critics: they desire our blood, not our pain.* Maybe it doesn't hurt to distance ourselves from our own work and consider each critic's motivation and point of view.

And what about a critic's special talents? Confucius said, *There is no one who does not eat and drink, but few are those who can distinguish flavors.* Now, am I trying to flatter any potential big-city critics? Certainly not!

To me, the most-useful reviews I've gotten haven't been the ones that glow. Although my ego longs for the Toxic-Glowing kind, the rest of me values mixed reviews—and that's a good thing, since that's mostly what I get. I appreciate those critics who take the time to point out a positive or two and then challenge me to improve if I can. If we always got glowing reviews, wouldn't we become altogether complacent? Give me a critic who cares to gently better me instead!

The best critics of all have not been professional reviewers. They are people like you. Mark Twain said, *The public is the only critic whose opinion is worth anything at all,* and I couldn't agree more.

CRITICISM AND THE BIG FLUFFY DUCK

Of course, criticism hurts even if you try not to let it. I drive myself crazy with just the fear of criticism. (Even as I write this, I wonder if I will be criticized for being too self-conscious or too simple or too something else. Or maybe not enough of this or that? Even worse, what if my work makes no impression at all? . . .)

I won't tell you how I know him or where he lives, but I got to speak to someone who's learned to handle mountains of criticism, "crazy mail," and even the occasional death threat. He's Bruce Tinsley, the creator of the very controversial Mallard Fillmore editorial comic strip, and he's developed a pretty healthy attitude about critics and criticism. (And now for another worry: Will Lost Souls with liberal leanings take me to task for learning something from a *conservative* cartoonist?)

King Features Syndicate has distributed Bruce's strip since 1994, and Mallard Fillmore now runs in about four hundred newspapers nationwide. Some people say it's the worst strip in the papers. Mallard is a fluffy, conservative duck that people either love or hate. A spokesperson for

Bruce's syndicate explained, "There's no in-between." Judging by his mail, Bruce would have to agree. He receives between forty and seventy letters a week, and they are rarely lukewarm.

Many letters are very positive. His fans say they are pleased that their points of view are finally being represented in the newspaper.

As for the rest of his mail? He said, "Some of the mail is really scary—the mail that threatens physical violence." But, he says, other letters bother him "almost as much as the death threats." He said, "It's one thing to say, 'You're completely wrong on this issue,' or 'You're a fascist,' but when somebody writes to me and says, 'You're not funny,' well, that really hurts! That does it." I suspect it's Bruce's sense of humor that gets him through most days.

A sense of professionalism helps too. "When I get a lot of [hate] mail . . . it's also a sign to me that I'm doing my job. You know one of the raps on newspapers today that really rings true is that they're boring, and I try to have a product that's exciting—even if you don't agree with it—and that stirs up debate," he said. Bruce says he never expected so many people to care on either side. I think it's pretty gratifying to him that they do.

He does offer this caveat about criticism: "For some reason there's always going to be a group of people out there . . . that gets its jollies out of tearing other people down. That doesn't mean that all criticism isn't valid. Some criticism that really hurts is nevertheless valid.

"At least in my case I get some of the worst from my wife. She's usually right when she says, 'This isn't particularly funny; you're forcing something here,' or when she'll say, 'This isn't fair to say this. This is going to hurt someone you didn't intend to hurt.' I think she's usually right."

As for all of the less constructive criticism, I think some of Bruce's early art instructors toughened him up for that. He postulates that some fine-art teachers, for example, are themselves frustrated or failed artists. As a result, instead of being supportive of students, they can be unusually cruel. (Those of you in art school will have to tell me if this sounds familiar.) "I think a lot of people are teaching for the very best reasons, but I think most of us have run into that teacher who'd rather be doing something else and compensates for it by tearing down students," Bruce explained.

Many of his art teachers disapproved of the fact that, as a student, Bruce created artwork for newspapers and ad agencies. He said, "They really felt like, you know, to be a real artist you had to starve and you couldn't make a profit from your artwork. [They thought that] in some sense I was being untrue to my craft. . . . [I was] doing violence to all artists and art in general by drawing stuff that sold a product. I was just trying to get through college! But I found there to be a really general kind of antipathy toward commercial art in the fine-arts field."

Bruce points out that professors have more power and influence than they may realize. "Professors [deal] with people at some of the most impressionable times of their lives, and they can really turn somebody off from a particular artistic field—forever. The things they say really mean a lot, and, for me, I think if I hadn't had the kind of affirmation of getting a paycheck from an ad agency or something it could've really affected me. You know, I could've felt like, *Gosh, you're right. I'm awful.*

"Oftentimes the best kind of counter to criticism is just to redouble your efforts and keep practicing and working and doing what you do."

Of course, you may never have bags and bags of hate mail to contend with, but the occasional negative comment or bad review is nearly unavoidable. I guess, like Bruce, we can always take comfort in the fact that we've gotten *some* sort of reaction from people. Whenever I fail to find value in criticism coming my way (which isn't very often, since I tend to believe most everything I hear), I do my best to just let it roll off me—like water off a duck's back.

WEAVE SOME POTHOLDERS, GO TO ROME, FILL YOUR TANK

When I *do* let things bother me too much, I become monumentally stuck. Those are the terrible times when I don't have anything to say, I don't feel much like drawing or painting, and if the earth opened up at my feet I would gladly throw myself in. Instead, I make potholders. They're each about three inches square, and I'm afraid they're all over the house. My roommate and I use them as coasters and bookmarks and doorstops, if we use them at all.

I used to make these potholders constantly when I was a kid. Back then it was just something to do, but now it is essential to my creative process. No, really. I use the same kind of loom as before—a red plastic one that comes with a *rustproof!* metal hook. (Multicolor cotton loops sold separately.) Like riding a bicycle or playing the drums, the task of creating scads of ugly potholders uses a different part of my brain, and I get to give everything else a rest. I make as many as I can stand, until I can't look another potholder in the face, and then I'm ready to get back to work.

I'm not telling you this so that you'll run out and start making potholders. Just know that doing something else for a while—especially something you can do on autopilot—can help you out of a creative slump.

If you're really, really stuck, you may have to do something drastic. My friend Paul and I saved up enough money to travel to Rome in the off-season, because we decided that maybe we needed to climb Mount Vesuvius. We didn't realize it at the time, but we were busy refilling our creative tanks.

Mark Twain coined the phrase, and he admitted that

sometimes it took him years to refill his tank. When he was working on *Tom Sawyer,* he got completely stuck by page 400. In Milton Meltzer's *Mark Twain Himself,* Twain described his own quandary, saying, *"I was disappointed, distressed and immeasurably astonished, for I knew quite well that the tale was not finished and I could not understand why I was not able to go on with it. The reason was very simple—my tank had run dry; it was empty; the stock of materials in it was exhausted; the story could not go on without materials; it could not be wrought out of nothing.*

"When the manuscript had lain in a pigeonhole two years I took it out one day and read the last chapter that I had written. It was then that I made the great discovery that when the tank runs dry you've only to leave it alone and it will fill up again in time, while you are asleep—also while you are at work on other things and are quite unaware that this unconscious and profitable cerebration is going on."

I guess I'd better mention that tank refilling and normal procrastination are not the same thing. The tank refill is your handsome brain taking a brisk walk as opposed to staring at its belly button.

Tanks run dry all the time. I think it's just part of the creative process for some of us. It doesn't hurt to give your creative tank time to refill. Do something else until you feel strong enough to return to your work with renewed passion. You might try digging in a garden or cleaning out your closets if climbing Vesuvius isn't an option just now. And please don't worry. Great things will come to you again.

A LITTLE SOMETHING HOPEFUL

If you read my first book, you met a character named Michael Teague, a painter/comix artist who has consistently chosen underemployment in order to have the time to devote to his creative work. Although he's in his mid-forties, Michael lives like a student—in a single rented sleeping room. He shares a bathroom with several other renters, and he cooks simple meals in his room. Now his sacrifice and persistence are finally paying off.

For one thing, he's scheduled to exhibit some of his new paintings in a Los Angeles gallery. Also, he received a grant from the Xeric Foundation and released his first comic book called *Epic Dermis Part 1*. You may remember his comic "Second Chance," featuring the Glitter Glue Fairy, from *The Lost Soul Companion*. Now you can enjoy Paint-by-Numbers Orphan Girl in "Hopeful," which Michael made especially for *The Not-So-Lost Soul Companion*.

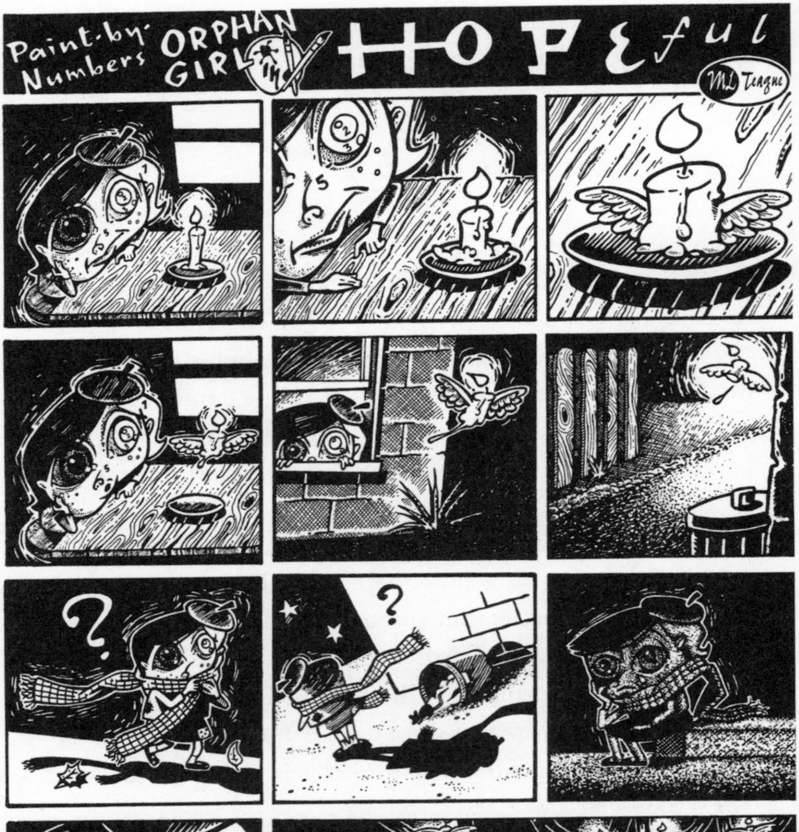
Paint-by-Numbers ORPHAN GIRL
HOPEful
ML Teague
?
?
!
THE END

yay
&
hooray!

THE CUTTERS AND THE "BIG DEAL"

There is a continuum that I think about a lot. It looks like this:

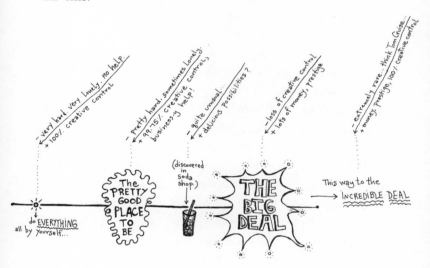

Many creative Lost (and even Not-So-Lost) Souls may find themselves squarely hoping and praying for that right side—the Big Deal with a record label or book publisher or New York art gallery. But that side of things isn't necessarily the best place to be.

There are plenty of advantages to the Big Deal, but there are several disadvantages too. There's a really nice guy named Rob Calder who knows a good deal about the Big Deal. He's the bass player for a band called The Cutters, and he's been at each end of that continuum and many points in between. He may or may not realize this, but I believe he has developed a very workable plan for true success.

The Cutters are four friends who've been playing together since 1993. They've recorded at A&M Records' studios; their music has been featured on MTV's *Undressed;* and they've even landed a record deal with CMC International. Nevertheless, there are plenty of things Rob and his bandmates wish they'd done differently. He explained, "Early on I read a lot of books [for musicians]. People would say, 'Just make a four-song demo. It doesn't need to be high quality. All we need to do is hear the songs, and if the songs are good, fine.' " So for years the band made hundreds of demos instead of releasing full-length CDs. They mailed them out blindly and, according to Rob, "One of them ended up on the proper desk of an A&R guy at A&M Records. Over the phone he just invited me and the rest of the guys out to Los Angeles to record for a week in their studio. It was just blind luck. We almost didn't believe it."

They asked the guy to at least send them something so they knew this was a legitimate deal. He sent them something, all right.

"He took this piece of paper and he wadded it up really

tightly and he taped it with duct tape and he put it in an envelope. You open it up and it said something like, *You suck . . . The Nixons sux.*

(They were called the Nixons before they became the Cutters, you see...)

You bring your instruments, and I'll provide the beer. But it was all on A&M letterhead. We blindly bought the plane tickets and flew out there and it ended up being a fantastic experience."

The bad news is that the A&R guy was fired and the deal fell through. Unfortunately, this sort of thing happens a lot. There's even a phrase for it: being orphaned. Rob remembered, "We ended up talking to the engineer that did the recording session just about a half a year ago and he admitted that we were going to be signed—just like we had feared—but that this guy ended up getting fired."

After the A&M disappointment, The Cutters decided to change their strategy. "[We thought], okay, we've done enough demos. We're going to make something ourselves, and we're going to sell it on our own and hope we can get some attention with the sales. So we made a full record and it was somehow taken more seriously because it was a full record and not a demo. We did the typical business things. We put a bar code on it. We [formed] a record company called Green Van Records."

The homegrown label released a new Cutters album, *Sonic Wave Love,* and then something really cool happened.

"This is a great, weird story," Rob said. "Tommy, the lead

singer, his dad bought some condominiums down in Naples as investments and he contacted just a regular real-estate agent: Over the years, every time we would do a little tape or something that wasn't a CD—just something casual—Tom Senior would give his real-estate agent the tapes. So when *Sonic Wave Love* came out, he gave him a CD. He said, 'Here you go. Check it out.'

"The real-estate agent listened to the CD and was blown away by it. He was just absolutely floored. He ended up forming an office without even talking to us. He wanted to become a band manager, and he decided that he was going to solicit us to be our manager, to get us going to where we needed to be. We said, 'Okay. That's great. We'll do it.'

"He downsized his job in terms of how much he was doing. He still works as a real-estate agent, but if you were to ask him he would say that he mainly works on The Cutters now. He was earning a lot of money and just kind of set that all aside. He ended up getting us signed."

Sonic Wave Love was rereleased by CMC International. (I love that The Cutters believed enough in their abilities as a band to make some sacrifices and release their own album. It just goes to show that once you demonstrate that you believe in yourself and your project, sooner or later others will too!) Still, the story doesn't really end here. . . .

CMC ended up merging with another record company and they dropped all of their new bands—including The Cutters—but not before Rob and the others learned that the coveted Big Deal can be rather vexing.

Maybe it's just because I'm from the Midwest, but it looks like some big companies exhibit a stunning lack of common sense. According to Rob, CMC had spent lots of money on marketing and promotion, but they didn't sensibly coordinate their efforts. He explained, "There was a radio station in Richmond, Virginia, that we were being played on a lot and very visibly. They were announcing us, and it was the perfect scenario for us.

"When we went and played there, we had a fantastic response. And then somebody said, 'Hey, when can we get your CD?' 'Well, you know, it should be in the store.' 'Well, it's not!' So we went and we started looking in all the stores, and our CD was nowhere to be found. Or they had one CD over at that place and it was long gone and sold. The record company never made the connection to put the CDs where there was radio play. They just scattered it out there in various places.

"And the record company would say, 'Hey, guys, you know we're getting a lot of radio play there in Richmond, but we're not getting any sales. What's going on, guys?' And they would hold that to us. 'Hey, this isn't working out very well, guys.' "

The same thing happened to them in Florida. Lots of airplay, but no CDs in the local stores. The Cutters tried to explain the situation to the label, with no results. Finally the

Cutters' manager took a box of CDs to the music stores himself. The stores were happy to have them, but, as Rob explained, "The record label and the distribution company got furious because [our manager] undermined them and their system. What was a no-brainer became a bad situation all the way around."

Certainly, there are benefits to being your own boss. "When I look at working with a major record label, that is a headache. That's the plus when you're in Green Van Records. When something needs to be done, you do it. There's no question about it. . . . Also, you're not going to give up on yourself, as is always a possibility if you're working with a major label. They could just as easily say, 'Okay. We're done.' And stop at any time."

On the other hand, having an established record label's backing can make some things much easier. Rob explained, "It's really hard as Green Van Records to get a song played on the radio. So in some sense it's a terrible Catch-22. There's only so much you can do as Green Van Records." True, but there's still a lot to be said for doing things yourself.

The Cutters hope that Green Van Records will be a vehicle to get them to their next Big Deal, but even if nothing happens for a very long time, they can survive indefinitely in the near-perfect balance between retaining creative control, juggling the inevitable business-y details, and feeling confident that common sense is being employed. Sure, you could be at the far left (or even the far right!) end of the continuum, but I still think inching over to the middle is every artist's best bet.

THE WIZARD BEHIND THE CURTAIN

I've still never seen *The Wizard of Oz* all the way through. For some reason, every time I try to watch it I fall asleep shortly after the beginning of the movie. But I am aware that the "wizard" is revealed in the end.

God knows I'm always craning my neck to steal a peek at whatever it is I'm not supposed to see. Naturally the fact that I have a working relationship with a traditional publishing house fascinates me. I am taking it all in quickly in the event that someone closes the curtain.

So far I've managed to glimpse good things and bad. It was exciting to see so many people—with Random House–sized resources at their disposal!—who believed in my project. There were editors and designers and an entire marketing staff having the occasional meeting about something that used to exist only in my own head.

But with the involvement of others comes the inevitable need for compromise. I did lose a little creative control, but, as I am not the literary equivalent of Metallica, that was to be expected. I think it wasn't nearly as bad as it could've been. There were only two big changes that I despaired over briefly. One was the cover art, and the other was the book's subtitle.

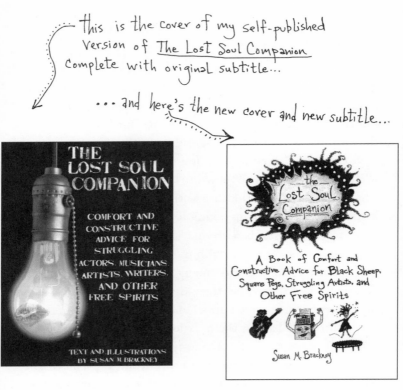

This is the cover of my self-published version of *The Lost Soul Companion* complete with original subtitle...

... and here's the new cover and new subtitle...

The publishers thought my original cover looked too depressing, and they asked me to do some sketches to replace it. (I tried to tell them that I'd hoped to attract Lost Souls with a dark image they could relate to, but ultimately I thought I'd better just shut up.) As it turns out, lots of people have told me they like the new cover much better than the old one, so that's good. In little doses, creative compromise isn't all bad.

But many writers with book deals aren't nearly so lucky! I met a woman who told me that her publisher changed her book's title and came up with cover art without ever consulting her. She cried when she saw it.

Why am I telling you all this? Because if and when other people *do* validate your work—for instance, if your band gets signed to a record label or your first novel's going to press or maybe your paintings are picked up by a big gallery—you may have notions of how things will turn out, but you'll hardly ever guess right. I just want you to be prepared to be occasionally disappointed, a little perplexed, excited, and happy, and a hundred other things too.

LEARNING FROM THE LISA-PEOPLE

I will always believe that starting small, having realistic goals, and doing as much on your own as you can is the best strategy to feel happy and accomplished. Add good Lisa-people to that mix, and now you've really got something. . . .

My friend Lisa is a freelance writer who lives by her wits. She's the sort of person who makes you think all things are possible, so when she asked me to share her office space, I was naturally delighted.

Our office was a small room above an Afghan restaurant, and there were massage therapists on either side of us. The faint smell of patchouli incense and the moaning of naked people didn't do much for my writing, but being around Lisa made up for that. First of all, she has beautiful, squiggly hair and a quick smile that I like, but, better still, she is very good at engineering her own success.

She is so daring in this regard that she once moved to New York City based on a picture of a lady in a magazine. Lisa explained, "[The lady in the picture was] standing in Central Park, and she had on a neat little suit. She's got the old-style Apple laptop and it's open and she's biting it! The caption is *Byte Me.* It was this article about women's websites. . . . I decided I was going to work for her. I did not know when. I didn't know how. But I truly had a vision, and I just decided that she would be someone I'd work for. I tore the magazine page out and carried it around with me."

Even though she'd been accepted to two grad schools and she'd agreed to a teaching-assistant position in San Diego, she radically changed course when a friend in New York called to say she had an extra room for rent. Lisa recalled, "[The rent there would be] $680 for my share, and here I was paying $320. . . . That was more than double my rent!

"But . . . on one coast it was all planned out. The next three years I would get a job and I would go to school and I

162

would be a TA and I would maybe live on the beach. . . . I could see it too clearly. And in New York—no job, no money. I went there with fifteen hundred dollars. No Web experience. No editorial experience. But a vision. And hope. And craziness. It seemed so much more exciting to me. . . . Going and failing would've been better than just going through the next three years and living my little existence. And I kept asking myself, where do I want to spend the main part of my twenties—the really good parts? . . . Where do I want to spend my youth and energy?"

She started working on her third day there, temping for *Reader's Digest,* and, yes, eventually she finagled a meeting with the woman in the photo and her staff. Lisa recalled, "I told them, 'You don't realize it, but I moved out here to work for you.' And they were blown away. They're a small company, and the CEO likes risk takers." Lisa convinced the company that (1) they needed to create an editorial position that had not previously existed, and (2) she was clearly the best pick for the job.

Of course, you know that sometimes we work and work for whatever it is we think we want, only to find that we don't like it nearly as much as we thought we would. After six months in the editing job she created for herself, Lisa realized she wasn't as happy as she thought she'd be. No problem. She left New York, but she kept working for the woman in the photo—this time on a freelance basis. And she finally knew what she really wanted to be: not a full-time editor but a freelance writer instead.

Lisa's ability to change her own circumstances reminds me of the plastic surgery shows I've seen on TV. I once watched a surgeon reshape a piece of this girl's hipbone to make her a new lower jaw like it was nothing. But it *is* a messy job that requires serious skill and a steady hand. The same is true for Lisa. I've seen the messy parts: Sometimes she stretches out on the floor of our little office and just cries and cries because she doesn't know where her next bit of freelance work will come from. But she always collects herself eventually and manages to figure something out. (That's her skill and steady hand coming through.)

If you haven't come across any Lisa-people yet, I hope you do soon. They won't all be named Lisa, but they can be indispensable to Lost Souls, since they are the kind of people who will encourage us even when no one else does.

Here are some of the very best things I've learned from my **Lisa-person...**

1. Always show up.

"A smile and a good attitude go a long way. Truthfully—for nearly half of life—it's just showing up. . . . Sometimes it's just a matter of

164

being in the right place at the right time and talking
to people."

2. Have a plan.
"I think when you have a plan, it really brings things
into focus. Those things have always been there, but
either you don't see them or you don't seek them out.
Suddenly it's just like putting on a pair of glasses and
things make sense."

3. Never be afraid to ask for what you want.
"When I was a telemarketer, I learned how to sell somebody on something in, like, five seconds. . . . I became
assertive. You should at least give the person an opportunity to say no. You never know."

4. You'll be surprised who will support you.
"It's kind of like moving day. . . . When it comes time
to move, you're always surprised who shows up [to
help] and who doesn't."

5. Be open to anything.
"On the surface, not every opportunity might look like
it relates to your future, but it can. You have to be sure
to learn something every time. Whether you are a de-
livery driver, whether you're a bartender, whether you
have some shit job where you have to mow or rake leaves

. . . there is something in that that you can take away that will help you with your next thing. . . . Make sure that there's more value to [your job] than just your paycheck. There's more to learn. And it will help whether you're trying to sell your art or you're trying to sell your stories or your music or your business or whatever."

As it turns out, Lisa even has Lisa-people of her own! She says the constant encouragement of other risk takers gets her through the rough spots. "I like people who go for it. I look for people that are following some voice or vision of theirs. People who are guided by something else—it's those people I treasure. It's those people that make life interesting. It's those folks who I rely on a lot."

And, who knows, maybe she'd have trouble sustaining her Lisa-ness without them. If you think that you could be a Lisa-person for someone else, by all means do!

CREATIVE SALONS

In addition to Lisa-people, some members of your own family may offer encouragement and inspiration just when you need it. In my case, my mom and dad are just happy that I'm still alive, so I don't have to do too much to please them. They've always encouraged me in my creative pursuits, because they know that my writing and doodling make me happy. Not everyone is nearly so lucky. Your family members may not fully understand why you steal every bit of spare time to write or paint or act. . . . Maybe you are the creative mind that Pearl S. Buck describes here:

For the truly creative mind in any field is no more than this—a human creature born abnormally, inhumanly sensitive. To him a touch is a blow, a sound is a noise, a misfortune is a tragedy, a joy is an ecstasy, a friend is a lover, a lover is a god, and failure is death. Add to this cruelly delicate organism the overpowering necessity to create—to create—to create— so that without the creating of music or poetry or books or buildings or something of beauty and meaning his very breath is cut off from him. He must create. He must pour out creation. By some strange unknown pressing inward urgency he is not really alive unless he is creating.

Sound familiar? Some people don't feel alive unless they're watching TV. For others, it's kayaking. Everyone has his thing. It just happens that the life of an artist is a little harder to explain. Your family may not relate to you, but they probably love you just the same. It's okay if you don't have their support; you can seek support for your creative work elsewhere. Why not assemble a "family" of your own once or twice a month? (But, remember, your new "family" shouldn't serve as a replacement for your real one unless your real one's burning you with cigarettes or something.)

Some old friends of mine used to host modern-day salons at their art gallery/apartment space. I would ride my bike over right after I finished my crappy telemarketing job around nine P.M. every Thursday night and enter a magical space filled with delectable food and very inspiring people. They were a shifting bunch, but at the core were a couple of videographers—local celebrities, really—writers, artists, a photographer or two. Sometimes there were discussion topics and sometimes not. Sometimes it was as pretentious as it sounds, but usually it was energizing.

Like minds used to gather themselves and talk about their creative pursuits all the time. When Gertrude Stein moved to Paris, she and her companion, Alice B. Toklas, regularly hosted all sorts of interesting people, including Ernest Hemingway, Picasso, Matisse, Ezra Pound, Sherwood Anderson, and F. Scott Fitzgerald. (Not that *we* were nearly as sophisticated and accomplished as these heavy hitters, mind you. . . .)

Salons don't have to be nearly so complicated. You can meet a few other musicians or illustrators or whomever you like for coffee occasionally. You don't even have to call them "salons." No, if "salons" sounds too pretentious for you, you can simply call them "get-togethers." (Of course, if "salons" isn't pretentious enough, you can call them "Meetings of Future Great Minds.") If you don't know many creative souls, why not put a classified ad in your local daily or an alternative weekly? Or tack up a couple of signs. Then go to your designated spot and wait to see who shows up. . . . Exciting!

A NOD TO THE BEHIND-THE-SCENES PEOPLE

My biggest pet peeves: toothpaste squeezed in the middle, those rude NASCAR decals, and the terrible twin myths of "overnight success" and "self-made" celebrity. Why do so many people believe that their favorite artists were able to reach the very stars all by themselves? Maybe it's too many issues of *People* magazine or *Entertainment Weekly*. Maybe people just desperately want the stories to be true.

The whole truth is that many well-known actors, painters, and writers, for instance, had plenty of quiet supporters—mothers and fathers, husbands and wives, patrons and mentors—behind the scenes, pulling the levers to help them fly. I wanted to honor them somehow (and remind you that it's perfectly okay to need help sometimes), so I decided to make a decent list of them.

It was my dad who gave me the idea for this chapter. He ought to know about being supportive. He's the one behind my mother and me—driving us to art fairs, helping set up our art displays, bringing us snacks while we're rooted to the spot, selling our wares. He tells us what he honestly thinks of our creative work, and he helps us in hundreds of other ways too. We are better artists and better people for having him in our lives.

Of course, I thought that compiling my Supportive-People-Behind-the-Famous-People type of list might be a little tricky. When you think about the value we place on inner strength, self-reliance, and, yes, fame, it makes sense that there wouldn't be much information on the selfless contributions of relatively obscure people. As it turns out, I might as well have been looking for the Tooth Fairy's second cousins. Regardless, I managed. These people aren't necessarily household names, but their efforts certainly helped to create a few. . . .

Behind Great Painters...

Paul Gachet was a doctor in Paris who treated Impressionist artists Pissarro, van Gogh, and Cézanne in exchange for their sketches and paintings. (Would any living doctor do such a thing today?) To amass still more art, he made a special house call for Renoir and once lent money to Monet. The doctor also treated musicians and actors in exchange for tickets to their performances.

Even though he didn't have a lot of money, Victor Chocquet, a French customs agent, also collected the work of Renoir and Cezanne, and a French pastry chef named Eugene Murer was very supportive of the circle of Impressionist artists as well.

Now, if you still live with your parents and you're over thirty, take comfort. Some of the Impressionist painters lived with their parents or stayed with other relatives. (Also, some painters simply lived off their parents' money indefinitely, but I don't advocate that.)

Finally, even though I wrote about him in my first book, it would be wrong of me not to mention Vincent van Gogh's brother, Theo, at least briefly. Offering unconditional emotional and financial support, Theo van Gogh was devoted to Vincent despite his own frailties and commitments. Because

Theo tirelessly promoted his brother's art, Vincent's work endures.

• • •

Lee Krasner, herself a painter, married abstract artist Jackson Pollock in 1945 and did everything she could to help advance his painting career. *Jackson Pollock* author Deborah Solomon writes, *Such was Lee's devotion to Pollock's career that she had no time or patience for people who couldn't help him get ahead.* Krasner did her best to organize the financial resources, entertain collectors and art dealers, and contain Pollock's alcoholism. (In return, Pollock was abusive and controlling, but that's another story entirely.)

The extensive financial support of Peggy Guggenheim—an art collector and gallery owner—enabled Pollock to paint full-time, and Thomas Hart Benton, one of Pollock's teachers, was so impressed with Pollock's abilities that he encouraged him for more than twenty years.

• • •

We might not know of Georgia O'Keeffe at all were it not for her friend Anita Pollitzer and Alfred Stieglitz (the man O'Keeffe eventually married). As the story goes, Pollitzer spirited away some of O'Keeffe's work to show to Stieglitz, who owned the 291 Gallery in New York. He liked what he saw and began showing O'Keeffe's work at the gallery. After the two were married, Stieglitz continued to help his reclusive wife by managing the business and public-relations aspects of her career.

Behind Great Composers...

Some say Robert Schumann's work wouldn't have had its staying power without his wife. Clara Schumann was herself a composer and a brilliant pianist. (She was a child prodigy, in fact.) She used her musical gift to promote her husband's compositions as well as those of Johannes Brahms. Of Clara's devotion to her husband's work, biographer Nancy B. Reich, in her book *Clara Schumann: The Artist and the Woman,* writes: *She considered it not only her sacred duty to play his music but her sacred right, and was jealous if his music was played by another pianist, anywhere.* A year after Robert's death in 1856, Clara moved to Berlin, where she continued to honor her husband's memory for many years.

• • •

For thirteen years, a wealthy widow named Nadezhda von Meck financially supported the composer Pyotr Ilich Tchaikovsky. At von Meck's request, the two never officially met. Von Meck encouraged other composers, including Claude Debussy, but I think Tchaikovsky was probably her favorite.

Behind Great Writers...

If your passion is writing, then you probably already know that a discouraged Stephen King gave up and tossed his unfinished draft of *Carrie* in the trash. His wife, Tabitha, fished it out. In *On Writing: A Memoir of the Craft,* King says, *I couldn't see wasting two weeks, maybe even a month, creating a novella I didn't like and wouldn't be able to sell. . . . The next night, when I came home from school, Tabby had the pages. She'd spied them while emptying my wastebasket, had shaken the cigarette ashes off the crumpled balls of paper, smoothed them out, and sat down to read them. She wanted me to go on with it, she said. She wanted to know the rest of the story.* King's wife told him, "You've got something here." Indeed he did. Doubleday eventually accepted *Carrie,* and Stephen King's writing career took off.

But long before he met and married Tabby, Stephen's mother, Ruth, was the one who encouraged him to write. When he was a small boy, she paid him a quarter each for four copies of one of his first short stories. King remembers, "That was the first buck I made in this business." More important, his mother told him that his writing was "good enough to be in a book." King continues, "Nothing anyone has said to me since has made me feel any happier."

• • •

The poet Gwendolyn Brooks was the first African-American to win the Pulitzer Prize for literature. In part, she owed her success to the encouragement of her mother and to writers James Weldon Johnson and Langston Hughes. Brooks loved to read the work of Paul Laurence Dunbar, and her mother often told her that she could be "the *lady* Paul Laurence Dunbar" if she liked. When she was just sixteen, Brooks sent some of her poems to Johnston and Hughes, who continued to encourage her. In particular, she became good friends with Hughes. (Interestingly, Hughes himself had a literary patron—an elderly white woman named Charlotte Mason who preferred to support him anonymously.)

Behind Garbo...

Greta Gustafsson's father told her that she could be famous someday. Despite his alcoholism and the family's extreme poverty, Karl Gustafsson often took Greta to buy candy and *magazines full of photographs of theatrical and film actresses at Agnes Lind's tobacco shop. He always let her have all the magazines she wanted, which meant as many as she could carry,* according to *Garbo* author Antoni Gronowicz. *Sometimes he hadn't enough money to pay for their purchases, and he would make an arrangement with the shopkeeper to pay for them the next day, saying to Greta, "Don't deprive yourself of things you would like to do or enjoy. Who knows, you might find your real future in them."*

She was devastated by his death in 1920 and fought bitterly with her mother, who did not support her acting dream. Just a few years later Greta Gustafsson would become Greta Garbo under the direction of Mauritz Stiller, a Swedish filmmaker and a kind of surrogate father to Greta. Without Stiller's connections and care, we might never have known a Greta Garbo at all.

• • •

You've probably already figured out that I would be honored to be one of the supportive people behind *you*. I'd like to be what a lady from Nigeria was for me. She had the smoothest brown skin and a high forehead. She wore her hair in long braids. She was one of those strangers you meet who make a lasting impression.

Her words struck me the most. She had a melodic way of speaking, and her voice reminded me of a xylophone. Someone had told her about *The Lost Soul Companion* project, and she said to me, "More grease to your elbows!"

She explained that it means that you wish someone success—or continued success—in whatever they do. This also happens to be my wish for you.

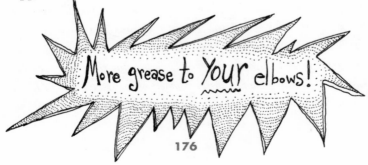

Now What?

You may be at the end of this book, but maybe you are at the beginning of something Wonderful. It is a fine time to start something Great (or to just keep doing your own Great Things if you already have been). Great Things can be small, and each time you successfully complete some project or other, you get stronger as a creative soul. Thinking of what to do next gets easier and easier. At least I think it does. . . .

Still, in my case, I'm not *exactly* sure what's next for me. Maybe I'll look at my Map of Future Plans and pick something else now. Maybe I'll keep writing, but only if I have something to say.

For sure I'm in the market for an old Airstream trailer. One of those fat silver ones. And a tiny parcel of land in the country. I hope to adopt a greyhound and call him "Dr. Bonesley," although the name he actually answers to will probably be something dumb.

Also, there will be a few chickens. The fancy kind that look like Tina Turner and Phyllis Diller.

I hope it helps to know that there's someone in your corner—even if it is just me and some chickens. As long as I'm alive and as long as I have *most* of my marbles, I will continue to offer you my well wishes and good vibes. You can send me snail-mail here and be assured of a hopeful reply.

> Susan M. Brackney
> The Lost Soul Companion Project
> P.O. Box 3248
> Bloomington, IN 47402-3248

Also, you can find other Lost Souls and more support on my Website at **www.lostsoulcompanion.com**. And there is this fantastic appendix for your enjoyment as well. . . .

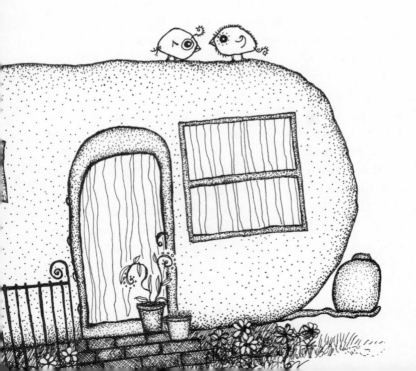

(the Appendix)

THE EXTRA BITS

After the debut of the self-published version of *The Lost Soul Companion,* lots of people wrote to ask me what ever happened to some of the different people I mentioned. You've already got the update on Michael Teague, but what of the others? For the most part they are happy. Not famous or rich. But at least satisfied and continuing to do the creative work that they love.

Well, everyone except for Steve. He's the musician-turned-law-student, and he's still in law school. The last time we spoke, I asked him what I should tell the people who were asking about him.

"People are asking about me?"
"Yes."
"No way."
"Yes way."

He joked around and told me to tell you that he got expelled and that they had to send him to a state mental hospital. But the truth is he recently made the dean's list.

• • •

Now, my friend Bill Robertson—the guy who reanimated Dazey the cow—has moved to Bisbee, Arizona, where he is known as "Road Kill Bill." Before he left Indiana, he finished work on a new road kill video called "A Road Kill Cautionary Tale," which made it all the way to the LA International Short Film Festival. *LA Weekly* said his was *undoubtedly . . . among the worst works of the festival.*

More recently, Bill acquired a dead horse, which he plans to do something interesting with.

• • •

Benjamin—the one who gave us blender food (plenty of sustenance with no tedious chewing)—says he's still afraid of his own artistic shadow. He continues to write songs and perform publicly now and then, but not actually as much as he should. An independent label is planning to rerelease one of his albums, but he doesn't know exactly when that will be.

• • •

Finally, there is Paul—my writer friend who tried to use a glass cutting board and a wax pencil to record his thoughts while in his bubble bath. He has hit upon something perfect: a small, plastic noteboard and special pencil used by scuba divers to communicate underwater. To get rid of old notes, he has to scrub them off with Comet and a brush. So that's turned out well, at least.

THE EXTRA EXTRA BITS

Here are a few more technical suggestions that didn't fit properly anywhere else:

One good way to protect your intellectual property is to keep a notebook. Be sure to date every entry, record whom you spoke with, and note what your conversation was about. (Something like *May 3, 1990—spoke by telephone to Philip Potts of the Exquisite Gallery. He offered me a one-woman show in the fall. He wants fifty percent of all sales.*) You can choose to have your notebook notarized, and if you ever have a legal problem, your notebook should be admissible in court.

• • •

Always keep a notebook and a good pen by your bed. The perfect plot twist could sneak into your dreams. Or the bass line that must back that new song you've been struggling with. Don't let them escape! Maybe a pendulous, luminescent pear will hang over you in the night to inspire you as never before.

• • •

My friend Jeff annoys the hell out of everyone around him by writing *everything* down. If someone triggers an idea in him, he stops whatever he's doing to capture it on an index card. Otherwise, he says, ideas tend to disappear. He started out with a small box for his ideas; now he has one big pile that he's been plundering for years.

MISCELLANEOUS RESOURCES

COPYRIGHT

U.S. COPYRIGHT OFFICE
http://www.loc.gov/copyright/

A COPYRIGHT PRIMER FOR THE ARTS
(from the National Endowment for the Arts)
http://arts.endow.gov/artforms/Manage/Copyrightla.html

UNITED STATES PATENT AND TRADEMARK OFFICE
http://www.uspto.gov/

LEGAL

ART LAW ON THE INTERNET
http://www.hg.org/art.html

STARVING ARTISTS LAW
http://www.starvingartistslaw.com

Volunteer Lawyers for the Arts
One East 53rd St., 6th Floor
New York, NY 10022
Phone: (212) 319-2787, Ext. 9
E-mail: Vlany@vlany.org
http://www.vlany.org

Marketing

Modern Post Card
1675 Faraday Ave.
Carlsbad, CA 92008
Phone: (800) 959-8365
http://www.modernpostcard.com/

Miscellaneous

Camp Sark
P.O. Box 330039
San Francisco, CA 94133
http://www.campsark.com

Books for More Inspiration
Inspiration Sandwich: Stories to Inspire Our Creative Freedom
SARK Celestial Arts, 1992

Resources for Actors

Actors Equity
165 West 46th St.
New York, NY 10036

Phone: (212) 869-8530
Fax: (212) 719-9815
E-mail: info@actorsequity.org
http://www.actorsequity.org/home.html
Union for American actors and stage managers
Benefits include: wage/labor agreement negotiations, contract
    administration/enforcement

SCREEN ACTORS GUILD
National Office/Hollywood Office
5757 Wilshire Blvd.
Los Angeles, CA 90036-3600
Phone: (323) 954-1600
TTY/TTD: (323) 549-6648
Fax: (323) 549-6603
E-mail: saginfo@sag.org
http://www.sag.org

New York SAG Office
1515 Broadway, 44th Floor
New York, NY 10036
Phone: (212) 944-1030
TTY/TTD: (212) 944-6715
Fax: (212) 944-6774
E-mail: nypr@sag.org
http://www.sag.org/branches/new_york
Benefits include: contract enforcement, workshops, newsletters,
    casting showcases, pension/health plans, scholarships

BOOKS OF INTEREST FOR ACTORS

Audition
Michael Shurtleff, Bob Fosse
Bantam Books, 1980 & Players Press, 1984

A Challenge for the Actor
Uta Hagen
Scribner, 1991

*Getting the Part: Thirty-Three Professional Casting Directors Tell You
How to Get Work in Theater, Films, Commercials, and TV*
Judith Searle
Limelight Editions, 1995

How to Audition: For TV, Movies, Commercials, Plays, and Musicals
Gordon Hunt
HarperCollins, 1995

*How to Be a Working Actor: The Insider's Guide to Finding Jobs in
Theater, Film, and Television*
Mari Lyn Henry, Lynne Rogers
Watson-Guptill Publications, 2000

Respect for Acting
Uta Hagen, Haskel Frankel
Hungry Minds Inc., 1973

Secrets of Screen Acting
Patrick Tucker
Theater Arts Books, 1993

RESOURCES FOR ARTISTS

AMERICAN INSTITUTE OF GRAPHIC ARTS
164 Fifth Ave.
New York, NY 10010
Phone: (212) 807-1990

Fax: (212) 807-1799

E-mail: comments@aiga.org

http://www.aiga.org

Benefits include: credit card, member discounts, publications, health insurance, competitions, conferences, exhibitions

AMERICAN SOCIETY OF PORTRAIT ARTISTS

Phone: (800) 62-ASOPA

E-mail: info@asopa.com

http://www.asopa.com

Benefits include: journal, awards, library, on-line portfolios, member discounts, seminars, critique service

AMERICAN WATERCOLOR SOCIETY

47 Fifth Ave.

New York, NY 10003

http://www.watercolor-online.com/AWS/

Benefits include: juried exhibitions, newsletter, promotion, social events

ARTCALENDAR: THE BUSINESS MAGAZINE FOR VISUAL ARTISTS

P.O. Box 2675

Salisbury, MD 21802

Phone: (410) 749-9625

Fax: (410) 749-9626

E-mail: info@ArtCalendar.com

http://www.artcalendar.com

Offers comprehensive listing of professional opportunities for visual artists. Includes juried shows, grant information, and more

THE GLASS ART SOCIETY

1305 Fourth Ave., Suite 711

Seattle, WA 98101

Phone: (206) 382-1305
Fax: (206) 382-2630
E-mail: info@glassart.org
http://www.glassart.org
Benefits include: journal, newsletter, conferences, member discounts

GRAPHIC ARTISTS GUILD
90 John St., Suite 403
New York, NY 10038-3202
Phone: (800) 500-2672
Fax: (212) 791-0333
http://www.gag.org
Benefits include: handbook, health/disability insurance, newsletter, member's discount, marketing assistance

NATIONAL ACRYLIC PAINTERS' ASSOCIATION USA (NAPA USA)
2525 E. 5th St.
Long Beach, CA 90814
Phone: (310) 439-3276
E-mail: NAPAinformation@watercolor-online.com
http://www.watercolor-online.com/NAPA/index.shtml
American branch of British organization
Benefits include: exhibitions, awards, newsletter, promotional activities

NATIONAL SCULPTURE SOCIETY
237 Park Ave.
New York, NY 10017-3140
Phone: (212) 764-5645
http://www.nationalsculpture.com/
Benefits include: newsletter, juried exhibitions, member discounts, journal, health/dental/disability insurance (some restrictions)

BOOKS OF INTEREST FOR ARTISTS

*Artist to Artist: Inspiration and Advice from Visual Artists
    Past and Present*
Clint Brown (Editor)
Jackson Creek Press, 1998

*An Artist's Book of Inspiration: A Collection of Thoughts on Art,
    Artists, Creativity*
Astrid Fitzgerald (Editor)
Lindisfarne Books, 1996

Getting the Word Out: The Artist's Guide to Self Promotion
Editors of *Art Calendar* (Editor)
The Lyons Press, 1998

How to Keep a Sketchbook Journal
Claudia Nice
North Light Books, 2001

*How to Survive & Prosper as an Artist: Selling Yourself Without Sell-
    ing Your Soul*
Caroll Michels
Henry Holt, 1997

RESOURCES FOR CRAFTSMEN

AMERICAN CRAFT COUNCIL
72 Spring St.
New York, NY 10012-4019
Phone: (212) 274-0630
Fax: (212) 274-0650

E-mail: council@craftcouncil.org
http://www.craftcouncil.org/

ART AND CRAFT SHOWS ON THE NET
http://www.artandcraftshows.net/

THE CRAFTS REPORT MAGAZINE
P.O. Box 1992
Wilmington, DE 19899
Phone: (800) 777-7098
Fax: (302) 656-4894
http://www.craftsreport.com/

RESOURCES FOR DANCERS/CHOREOGRAPHERS

THE AMERICAN DANCE GUILD INC.
P.O. Box 2006, Lenox Hill Station
New York, NY 10021
Phone: (212) 932-2789
E-mail: Julia@americandanceguild.org
http://www.americandanceguild.org
Benefits include: conferences, publications

NATIONAL DANCE ASSOCIATION
1900 Association Dr.
Reston, VA 20191
Phone: (703) 476-3421
Fax: (703) 476-9527
E-mail: nda@aahperd.org
http://www.aahperd.org/nda/nda_main.html
Benefits include: journal, newsletter, conventions, workshops,
    choreography evaluation

BOOKS OF INTEREST FOR DANCERS

Advice for Dancers: Emotional Counsel and Practical Strategies
Linda H. Hamilton
Jossey-Bass, 1998

Conversations with Choreographers
Svetlana McLee Grody, Frank Rich, Dorothy Lister (Contributor)
Heinemann, 1996

Dancer's Foot Book
Terry L. Spilken
Princeton Book Co., 1990

Ear Training for the Body: A Dancer's Guide to Music
Katherine Teck
Princeton Book Co., 1994

High Kicks: The Essential Guide to Working as a Dancer
Donna Ross
A&C Black, 1999

RESOURCES FOR SONGWRITERS/MUSICIANS

AMERICAN FEDERATION OF MUSICIANS
1501 Broadway, Suite 600
New York, NY 10036-5599
Phone: (212) 869-1330
http://www.afm.org
Benefits include: member discounts, life/medical/liability/accident insurance, PPO/medical savings accounts (some restrictions), job-referral programs, banking services

AMERICAN SOCIETY OF COMPOSERS, AUTHORS AND PUBLISHERS (ASCAP)
One Lincoln Plaza
New York, NY 10023
Phone: (800) 952-7227
Fax: (212) 595-3276
E-mail: info@ascap.com
http://www.ascap.com
Benefits include: royalties collection, magazine, showcases, workshops, publications, liability/theft/loss/dental/medical/life/accident insurance, credit union, banking services

THE FREELANCE MUSICIANS' ASSOCIATION
240 Commissioners Rd. W., Unit G
London, Ontario N6J 1Y1
Canada
E-mail: fma@execulink.com
http://www.execulink.com/~swr/fma
Benefits include: newsletter, venue database, booking-referral program

MUSICIANS' INTELLECTUAL LAW & RESOURCES LINKS
http://www.aracnet.com/~schornj/index.shtml

MUSIC VIDEO PRODUCTION ASSOCIATION
940 North Orange Dr., #104
Hollywood, CA 90038
Phone: (323) 469-9494
Fax: (323) 469-9445
E-mail: Musivideo@aol.com
http://www.mvpa.com
Benefits include: awards, newsletter, seminars, festivals

BOOKS OF INTEREST FOR SONGWRITERS/MUSICIANS

6 Steps to Songwriting Success: Comprehensive Guide to Writing and Marketing Hit Songs
Jason Blume
Watson-Guptill Publications, 1999

88 Songwriting Wrongs & How to Right Them: Concrete Ways to Improve Your Songwriting and Make Your Songs More Marketable
Pat Luboff, Pete Luboff (Contributor)
Writer's Digest Books; F&W Publications, Inc., 1992

How to Get a Job in the Music and Recording Industry
Keith Hatschek
Hal Leonard Publishing Corporation, 2001

The Independent Musician's Contact Bible
David Wimble
Big Meteor Publishing, 2000

The Musical Life: Reflections on What It Is and How to Live It
W. A. Mathieu
Shambhala Publications, 1994

The Musician's Survival Manual: A Guide to Preventing and Treating Injuries in Instrumentalists
Richard Norris, M.D.
MMB Music, 1993
(out of print)

RESOURCES FOR WRITERS

THE ACADEMY OF AMERICAN POETS
588 Broadway, Suite 1203
New York, NY 10012-3210

Phone: (212) 274-0343
Fax: (212) 274-9427
E-mail: academy@poets.org
http://www.poets.org/index.cfm
Benefits include: discussion groups, member discounts, audio
    recordings, journal

AMERICAN SOCIETY OF JOURNALISTS AND AUTHORS
1501 Broadway, Suite 302
New York, NY 10036
Phone: (212) 997-0947
Fax: (212) 768-7414
E-mail: execdir@asja.org
http://www.asja.org/index9.php
Benefits include: Referral service, workshops, industry news,
    market information, members' discounts

EDITORIAL FREELANCERS ASSOCIATION
71 West 23rd St., Suite 1910
New York, NY 10010
Phone: (212) 929-5400
Fax: (212) 929-5439
E-mail: info@the-efa.org
http://www.the-efa.org
Benefits include: newsletter, job listings, legal services,
    health/dental/disability insurance

HORROR WRITERS ASSOCIATION
P.O. Box 50577
Palo Alto, CA 94303
E-mail: hwa@horror.org
http://www.horror.org
Benefits include: newsletter, market reports, mentoring, agent
    lists, awards

MYSTERY WRITERS OF AMERICA
17 East 47th St., 6th Floor
New York, NY 10017
Phone: (212) 888-8171
Fax: (212) 888-8107
E-mail: mwa_org@earthlink.net
http://www.mysterywriters.net
Benefits include: newsletter, awards, health insurance,
    symposia, conferences

NATIONAL WRITERS UNION
National Office (East)
113 University Pl., 6th Floor
New York, NY 10003
Phone: (212) 254-0279
Fax: (212) 254-0673
E-mail: nwu@nwu.org

National Office (West)
337 17th St., #101
Oakland, CA 94612
Phone: (510) 839-0110
Fax: (510) 839-6097
E-mail: nwu@nwu.org
http://www.nwu.org
Union for freelance writers
Benefits include: arbitration, health/dental insurance, job list-
    ings, contract advice

THE POETRY SOCIETY OF AMERICA
15 Gramercy Park
New York, NY 10003
Phone: (212) 254-9628

http://www.poetrysociety.org
Benefits include: competitions, seminars, journal, readings

ROMANCE WRITERS OF AMERICA
3707 FM 1960 West, Suite 555
Houston, TX 77068
Phone: (281) 440-6885
Benefits include: journals, reports, local chapters, annual conference, health insurance, contests, awards

SCIENCE FICTION AND FANTASY WRITERS OF AMERICA
P.O. Box 877
Chestertown, MD 21620
E-mail: execdir@sfwa.org
http://www.sfwa.org
Benefits include: grievance/complaints resolution, publications, agent lists, speakers' bureau, legal fund, library, market reports, awards

THE SOCIETY OF AMERICAN TRAVEL WRITERS
1500 Sunday Dr., Suite 102
Raleigh, NC 27607
Phone: (919) 787-5181
E-mail: shaw@satw.org
http://www.satw.org
Benefits include: medical/term life/dental insurance (most states), conventions, newsletter, awards, legal/tax/financial advice, member discounts

SOCIETY OF CHILDREN'S BOOK WRITERS AND ILLUSTRATORS
8271 Beverly Blvd.
Los Angeles, CA 90048
Phone: (323) 782-1010

Fax: (323) 782-1892
E-mail: scbwi@scbwi.org
http://www.scbwi.org
Benefits include: national and regional conferences, newsletter,
    grants, awards

WESTERN WRITERS OF AMERICA
Larry K. Brown
209 E. Iowa
Cheyenne, WY 82009
E-mail: membership@westernwriters.org
http://www.westernwriters.org
For writers of fiction and nonfiction dealing with the America West
Benefits include: awards, annual convention, journal

WRITERS GUILD OF AMERICA (EAST)
555 West 57th St., Suite 1230
New York, NY 10019
Phone: (212) 767-7800
Fax: (212) 582-1909
http://www.wgaeast.org

WRITERS GUILD OF AMERICA (WEST)
7000 West Third St.
Los Angeles, CA 90048
Phone: Southern California callers (323) 951-4000
        Others (800) 548-4532
http://www.wga.org
Membership composed predominantly of screenwriters for the
    motion picture and broadcast industries
Benefits include: legal and arbitration services, agent lists,
    newsletter

BOOKS OF INTEREST FOR WRITERS

The 38 Most Common Fiction Writing Mistakes
  (And How to Avoid Them)
Jack M. Bickham
Writer's Digest Books, 1997

The Chicago Manual of Style: The Essential Guide for Writers, Editors,
  and Publishers
John Grossman
University of Chicago Press, 1993

The Elements of Style
William Strunk Jr., et al.
Allyn & Bacon, 2000

How to Write a Damn Good Novel
James N. Frey
St. Martin's Press, 1987

How to Write a Damn Good Novel II: Advanced Techniques for Dra-
  matic Storytelling
James N. Frey
St. Martin's Press, 1994

In the Palm of Your Hand: The Poet's Portable Workshop
Steve Kowit
Tilbury House, 1995

Line by Line: How to Improve Your Own Writing
Claire Kehrwald Cook
Houghton Mifflin, 1986

On Writing: A Memoir of the Craft
Stephen King
Pocket Books, 2001

On Writing Well: The Classic Guide to Writing Nonfiction
William K. Zinsser
Harper Resource, 1998; Quill, 2001

A Poetry Handbook
Mary Oliver
Harvest Books, 1995

Walking on Alligators: A Book of Meditations for Writers
Susan Shaughnessy
Harper San Francisco, 1993

Word by Word: An Inspirational Look at the Craft of Writing
John Tullius
Triple Tree Publishing, 2000

Writers on Writing: Collected Essays from The New York Times
John Darnton
Times Books, 2001

Zen in the Art of Writing: Essays on Creativity
Ray Bradbury
Joshua Odell Editions, 1994; Bantam Books, 1992

INDEX

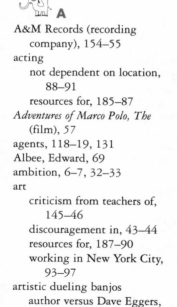

B

 C

PERMISSIONS